Peer Support in Medicine

Jonathan D. Avery
Editor

Peer Support in Medicine

A Quick Guide

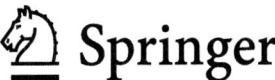

Editor
Jonathan D. Avery
Director of Addiction Psychiatry
Associate Professor of Clinical Psychiatry
Weill Cornell Medical College
New York, NY
USA

ISBN 978-3-030-58659-1   ISBN 978-3-030-58660-7 (eBook)
https://doi.org/10.1007/978-3-030-58660-7

© Springer Nature Switzerland AG 2021

This work is subject to copyright. All rights are reserved by the Publisher, whether the whole or part of the material is concerned, specifically the rights of translation, reprinting, reuse of illustrations, recitation, broadcasting, reproduction on microfilms or in any other physical way, and transmission or information storage and retrieval, electronic adaptation, computer software, or by similar or dissimilar methodology now known or hereafter developed.

The use of general descriptive names, registered names, trademarks, service marks, etc. in this publication does not imply, even in the absence of a specific statement, that such names are exempt from the relevant protective laws and regulations and therefore free for general use.

The publisher, the authors, and the editors are safe to assume that the advice and information in this book are believed to be true and accurate at the date of publication. Neither the publisher nor the authors or the editors give a warranty, expressed or implied, with respect to the material contained herein or for any errors or omissions that may have been made. The publisher remains neutral with regard to jurisdictional claims in published maps and institutional affiliations.

This Springer imprint is published by the registered company Springer Nature Switzerland AG

The registered company address is: Gewerbestrasse 11, 6330 Cham, Switzerland

Acknowledgment

Dr. Jonathan D. Avery would like to thank the Brause Family and the Brause Family Junior Faculty Assistance Award for supporting his work.

Introduction

Peer Support in Medicine: A Quick Guide is one of the only books that focuses on the use of peers to enhance medical care. This may come as a surprise, as the use of peers via trained peer specialists and in various individual and group settings has been one of the most important and meaningful developments in medicine over the last several decades. While initially different self-help and peer-led initiatives (such as alcoholics anonymous) were divorced from formal medical care, the evidence for their efficacy has increased, and medical professionals have embraced this additional way to help their patients. While there have been many studies looking at the efficacy of these peer-based interventions, there are few books on the topic. The primary goal of this book is to collect leading scholarly thought, providing both the clinician and the non-expert with a comprehensive understanding of the different aspects of the use of peers in medicine.

Chapter 1 covers peer support for substance use disorders, which is perhaps the best known use of peers in medicine. Peers though can be utilized to enhance the care of everyone, from adolescents (Chap. 5) to the elderly (Chap. 6) to even family members of individuals with medical and substance use disorders (Chap. 7). They can be especially helpful for individuals struggling with chronic medical (Chap. 3) and psychiatric (Chap. 2) illness. Peers often play an important role in bereavement (Chap. 4) as well. Just as I have, in discussing the chapters of this book, taken them topically and out of order, the reader should feel free to do the same. The chapters do not depend on one another, and they may be read in any order.

Jonathan D. Avery, M.D.

Contents

1. **Peer Support for Substance Use Disorders** 1
   Rachel N. Knight

2. **Peer Support for Mental Health** 31
   Ana Stefancic, Lauren Bochicchio, and
   Daniela Tuda

3. **Peer Support for Chronic Medical Conditions** 49
   Megan Evans, Timothy Daaleman, and
   Edwin B. Fisher

4. **Peer Support for the Bereaved** 71
   Paul T. Bartone and Chantel M. Dooley

5. **Peer Support for Adolescents with Chronic Illness** . . 95
   Yalinie Kulandaivelu and Sara Ahola Kohut

6. **Peer Support for Older Adults** 115
   Kimberly A. Van Orden and Julie Lutz

7. **Parent Peer Models for Families of Children
   with Mental Health Problems** 131
   Mary C. Acri, Emily Hamovitch,
   Anne Kuppinger, and Susan Burger

8. **Peer Support for the Medical Community** 145
   Beverly Shin

Index 181

Contributors

Mary C. Acri McSilver Institute for Poverty, Policy, and Research, New York, NY, USA

Department of Child and Adolescent Psychiatry, NYU Langone School of Medicine, New York, NY, USA

Paul T. Bartone Institute for National Strategic Studies, National Defense University, Washington, DC, USA

Lauren Bochicchio Columbia University School of Nursing, New York, NY, USA

Susan Burger Albany, NY, USA

Timothy Daaleman Department of Family Medicine, School of Medicine, University of North Carolina at Chapel Hill, Chapel Hill, NC, USA

Chantel M. Dooley Tragedy Assistance Program for Survivors, Arlington, VA, USA

Megan Evans Department of Health Behavior, Peers for Progress, Gillings School of Global Public Health, University of North Carolina at Chapel Hill, Chapel Hill, NC, USA

Edwin B. Fisher Department of Health Behavior, Peers for Progress, Gillings School of Global Public Health, University of North Carolina at Chapel Hill, Chapel Hill, NC, USA

Emily Hamovitch New York University, McSilver Institute for Poverty Policy and Research, New York, NY, USA

Rachel N. Knight New York-Presbyterian Hospital, Weill Cornell Medical Center, New York, NY, USA

Sara Ahola Kohut IBD Centre, The Hospital for Sick Children, Toronto, ON, Canada

Child Health Evaluative Sciences, SickKids Research Institute, Toronto, ON, USA

Department of Psychiatry, University of Toronto, Toronto, ON, Canada

Yalinie Kulandaivelu Institute of Health Policy, Management and Evaluation, University of Toronto, Toronto, ON, USA

Child Health Evaluative Sciences, SickKids Research Institute, Toronto, ON, USA

Anne Kuppinger NYU Child Study Center/IDEAS, Department of Child and Adolescent Psychiatry, New York, NY, USA

Julie Lutz Department of Psychiatry, University of Rochester School of Medicine & Dentistry, Rochester, NY, USA

Kimberly A. Van Orden Department of Psychiatry, University of Rochester School of Medicine & Dentistry, Rochester, NY, USA

Beverly Shin New York Presbyterian Hospital Weill Cornell Medicine, New York, NY, USA

Ana Stefancic Columbia University, Department of Psychiatry, New York, NY, USA

Daniela Tuda Columbia University, Department of Psychiatry, New York, NY, USA

Peer Support for Substance Use Disorders

Rachel N. Knight

Introduction

This is an exciting time in the history of addiction recovery. On a cultural and societal level, we are emerging from generations of personal shame and public stigma and entering into a space where individual recovery stories are not only encouraged but considered part of the solution to problematic substance use. One doesn't have to travel far to find some form of public display that encourages discourse on the topic of addiction. Recovery memoirs frequent bestsellers lists, and the narrative-style story of the impact of substance use is a rapidly growing genre in TV, film, music, theater, and podcasts. Celebrities and social media influencers use their associated platforms to discuss recovery and promote sober lifestyles, inspiring fans to contemplate their own relationship to drugs and alcohol. These public displays of personal struggle and resilience have tremendous power in connecting those who have been touched by addiction and may stimulate change for individuals with problematic substance use [34]. Those who derive meaning and promise from these stories are benefiting from a process

R. N. Knight (✉)
New York-Presbyterian Hospital, Weill Cornell Medical Center,
New York, NY, USA
e-mail: rnk9002@nyp.org

called mutuality. In the world of addiction, mutuality happens between peers – individuals who share experiential knowledge on a topic. As stigma decreases, we are seeing the increasing role that peers can play in recovery.

However, peer support is an underutilized resource in the current approach to substance use treatment which is traditionally delivered by clinical professionals. Peers have been informally tied to recovery for centuries in the context of mutual aid societies such as AA, but mutual support delivered by peers can be a salient component to a variety of different recovery pathways. Despite this, when clinicians think about the role of peer support in addiction, they will often recommend a 12-Step group like AA without knowing about the myriad of other mutual aid options or peer-support services (see Table 1.1 for basic definitions and an extended list of existing mutual aid societies, as well as non-mutual aid recovery resources that utilize peers). From a professional lens, peer work is considered a trusted but poorly understood

Table 1.1 Expanding on definitions

Terms and definitions
Peer support
The process of exchanging nonprofessional, nonclinical information between individuals who have similar conditions or experiences to achieve long-term recovery from substance-related problems [32]
Peer provider (examples include certified peer specialist, peer-support specialist, mentor, recovery coach)
A person who uses his or her lived experience of addiction and success in recovery plus skills learned in formal training to deliver services that promote comprehensive recovery [32]
Peer-based recovery support services
Services delivered by peers which are designed to fill the needs of people in or seeking recovery. They help enhance available clinical resources and extend into the community setting. These services help people become and stay engaged in the recovery process and reduce the likelihood of relapse (Center for Substance Abuse Treatment, What are Peer Recovery Support Services? [8])
Mutual aid
Nonprofessional support groups made up of members who share the same problem and voluntarily support one another in taking responsibility for that problem and in recovery from that problem [14]

Table 1.1 (continued)

Examples of mutual aid groups
12-Step groups (most common form of mutual aid)
Options include Alcoholics Anonymous (AA), Narcotics Anonymous (NA), Cocaine Anonymous (CA), Crystal Meth Anonymous (CMA), Pills Anonymous (PA), Alanon (family support group)
SMART Recovery
Women for Sobriety (WFS)
Secular Organizations for Sobriety/Save Our Selves (SOS)
Moderation Management
LifeRing Secular Recovery
American Atheists Alcohol Recovery Group [9]
Examples of non-mutual aid settings that may utilize peers
Sober homes
Residential treatment
Social setting detoxification
Methadone clinics
Therapeutic communities

component to the recovery process and is often siloed from clinically delivered treatment. Fortunately, as stigma recedes, we are beginning to break out of encapsulated categories of SUD treatment (professionally delivered care or mutual aid societies) and move toward a recovery-oriented system of care. Recently there has been a trend to broaden the scope of how peers are used in substance use treatment by using peer-based recovery services. These are distinct from the services offered by professionally directed care or other helping institutions like mutual aid. Instead they use peers in formal, specialized ways to provide a variety of support services tailored to the specific recovery stage and chosen recovery pathway (see Table 1.2 for the ways in which peer-based recovery services provide support and Table 1.3 for current examples where peer-based recovery services can function). In this chapter, I will provide an overview of the current approach to addiction treatment and examine some of the shortcomings. I will look at the history of mutual aid societies and show that they are a useful but singular approach to recovery and that there are other ways in which peers can be utilized meaningfully. The remainder of this chapter will focus on the existing research in the field of peer-based recovery support services to show how they have a

Table 1.2 Forms of support delivered by peers

Type of support	Description/example
Emotional	Combining empathy and concern with experiential knowledge to bolster an individual's self-esteem and hope surrounding achieving recovery. Can be delivered one-on-one through a personalized recovery coach, peer mentor, or peer-led support group
Informational/navigational	Recovery resource dissemination: connecting individuals to appropriate professional treatment, referrals to mutual aid or support groups, community resources, wellness seminars, vocational skills training
Instrumental	Concrete supports (to mitigate problems that often threaten engagement with recovery resources) like child care, transportation, help accessing health or community services
Affiliation	Helping to create a recovery community where a newly recovered individual feels they belong and can thrive: link to recovery community centers, sober social activities, sports leagues, local events that promote recovery education

Adapted from Center for Substance Abuse Treatment [8]

Table 1.3 Examples where peer-based recovery services are being used

Recovery community centers
Recovery residences
Drug courts/criminal justice settings
Hospital emergency rooms
Homeless shelters
Child welfare agencies
Behavioral health and primary care settings (inpatient and outpatient)
Detox facilities
Colleges and schools

unique potential to capture more individuals in need of treatment, improve treatment engagement, and support the framework for long-term recovery. Lastly, I will conclude with a brief discussion about the limitations to the current body of research and how the lack of formal definitions for how peers should be trained and applied presents a challenge to the field.

Overview

The Current Climate of Addiction Treatment

From a clinical, research, and policy perspective, there have been limited efforts to incorporate the firsthand knowledge from individuals in recovery into the existing professional approach to treating substance use disorders. Instead, treatment has historically been guided by evolving paradigms for understanding the etiology of addiction. Strategies like abstinence pledges or making drunkenness a punishable crime harken back to early beginnings where excessive substance use was understood as a character defect that could be resolved through will power. Since then, years of scientific research has led to the generally accepted idea that addiction is a legitimate health problem that warrants a medical approach to treatment. Acute, intensive medical interventions like detoxification and brief rehabilitation stays are helpful with temporary stabilization, but longitudinal studies have shown that these interventions are followed by high relapse rates and various cycles of treatment reentry. This has led to the notion that for many, addiction manifests itself like other chronic medical conditions. The current chronic care model combines acute medical treatment with long-term outpatient support services to help maintain desired behavioral changes, and evidence shows this approach helps individuals achieve reductions in their substance use and related problems.

Yet despite this advancement in understanding, we are still a society that struggles immensely with the impact of substance-related problems. There are about 20 million people with a substance use disorder (SUD) in the USA, and the prevalence has not changed substantially over the past decade [29]. This calls into question the effectiveness of current treatment approaches which emphasize pathology and acute stabilization. While clinical treatment has helped many enter into recovery, overall relapse rates for substance use disorders range between 40% and 60%. In addition, treatment doesn't reach the majority in need. In 2018, only 11% of people in need of treatment for a substance use disorder actually received it [29]. All of this demonstrates a significant void in the existing approach to the treatment of SUD.

There are a variety of different reasons why professional treatment models fall short. Treatment can be expensive and challenging to access. It lacks flexibility and is often not structured to support the tremendous variability inherent to each individual motivation for change and the factors that threaten recovery. Professional settings can be off-putting and lack a personalized approach; they are often laden with stigma, complex clinical language, and providers who, bound by professional considerations, are limited in their ability to form the deep therapeutic bonds essential to engaging someone in the process of recovery. While a modest proportion of individuals with lifetime substance dependence enter recovery at some point, there is great heterogeneity in this process. The majority of individuals who enter recovery do so by participating in clinical treatment, but others find success outside the confines of a formal treatment approach and rely heavily on informal institutions that fall under the category of mutual aid (with the most well-known example being 12-Step programs). Mutual aid programs emphasize the importance of social community and utilize peers – individuals who have shared lived experience – as a critical component to the recovery process. The process of initiating change, achieving, and maintaining longstanding recovery is a demanding process and one that clinical professionals often have a finite ability to relate to. Peers help mitigate this issue because they have lived experience in long-term recovery and possess valuable firsthand knowledge on the topic. For centuries mutual aid (and, therefore, peer support) has organically stepped in as an informal way of filling some of the voids inherent to formal treatment [10].

Brief History of Mutual Aid Societies

Organized mutual support has long-standing roots in the history of recovery. Cultural revitalization movements among Native American tribes led to the creation of sobriety support groups as a means to reject alcohol consumption – seen as a symbol for European cultural conquest. With the rise of the temperance movement in the 1800s, many people with drug and alcohol problems found refuge through a diverse array of mutual support groups. These groups were created by struggling alcoholics or drug users who were desperate to stay sober in a climate where problematic substance use had criminal and legal ramifications. Some of these groups were exclusively religious and promoted strict abstinence, while others were secular and utilized moderation-based frameworks. A shared notion between groups was that there was strength in solidarity, and relying on others who knew a similar struggle could inspire hope [36]. These original efforts seem to foreshadow an important concept that is becoming more clear in today's changing approach to addiction treatment: there is no single road to recovery, and there is wisdom to be learned from those on a similar journey [37].

Early models of mutual support set the stage for the creation of Alcoholics Anonymous (AA), founded in 1935 by a Bill W and Dr. Bob – a stockbroker and a physician who each utilized the other's story and support to reflect on their own alcoholism and stay sober. The 12 Steps are the backbone of AA and guide the process of achieving recovery. There are hundreds of thousands of groups across the USA; each one is autonomous and varies in the way the 12 Steps are discussed and applied. Some of the hallmarks of AA are the meetings (which can be open or closed and often involve discussing one of the 12 Steps), sponsorship (a mentor and role model who exemplifies how the program works), celebration of sobriety anniversaries, and the Serenity Prayer, which highlights the powerlessness of the individual over alcohol use [30]. Studies looking at the impact of AA show that the related benefits come from prescribed behaviors dictated by working the steps but also the social interaction inherent to attending meetings with peers [19].

Shortly after the birth of AA, new speciality groups utilizing 12-Step framework for people dependent on other drugs emerged (see Table 1.1 for examples). There have also been efforts to incorporate 12-Step principles into formal treatment settings, and some literature suggests that treatment programs who do may be more successful in promoting abstinence compared to those programs who do not use this framework [19]. However, there has been little investigation into the specific reasons this approach is useful, and it may be the case that the enhanced social connection and component of shared lived experience confers benefits, rather than the use of the 12-Step framework which happens to be readily accessible outside of these costly treatment venues, free of charge.

Success from 12-Step work seems to be correlated with meeting attendance, and most likely the individuals with consistent attendance are the ones that find this environment to be a good fit. This is to say that for the many who are helped by 12-Step programs, the rewards may be a reflection of their unique demographic, substance use patterns, and psychosocial circumstance. Individuals from minority groups often have more negative experiences in these types of programs, and the spiritual component of 12-Step can also be a deterrent for some. In addition, a core tenant of the work is admitting powerlessness to the forces of drug and alcohol. This notion can be uninviting and ultimately repelling for individuals who are simply looking to explore their relationship to substance use and initiate help without fully identifying as being an "addict" [39]. This may be why research has shown that those who seem to benefit most from something AA are individuals who have severe alcohol use and are committed to abstinence [19].

In the past 50 years, there has been a surge of alternative groups that diversify the menu of mutual aid options (see Table 1.1). SMART Recovery is one example. Different than AA or 12-Step, this is an evidence-based program that focuses on promoting tools for recovery through discussion-style forums. There are countless other alternatives that have emerged, often tailored to meet the needs of a specific demographic, life-stage, or personal circumstance. Despite this diversification, 12-Step continues to be the most readily available mutual aid modality across the nation and the one that is most frequently promoted by professionals. Physicians often lack familiarity with the nuances of these various nonclinical institutions and, as such, can fail to capitalize on the critical role they play as a potential facilitator to finding support resources.

Mutual aid can be an alternative to formal substance use treatment or an adjunct to professionally delivered care. Physicians commonly "prescribe" meetings to their patients who struggle with addiction. However, this process works best when the physician is well informed about the variety of options, the way these programs are structured and function, as well as when there are attempts to follow up on attendance [30]. For the busy clinician who may have a limited personal relationship to addiction or the nuances of recovery support groups, this ends up being an idealistic expectation instead of the norm. This exemplifies a long-standing problem in the culture of addiction treatment where the primary approach remains largely clinical and focused on pathology and intervention [35]. In turn, a focus on supporting recovery through the use of mutual aid modalities has often been treated like an afterthought to boost clinical care or as an entirely self-contained entity.

There have been efforts to break out of these distinct categories of mutual aid or professional treatment and enhance the approach to recovery. Halfway houses and therapeutic community models are excellent exceptions to the mold and attempt to blend some of the benefits of clinical and nonclinical institutions. While these programs are not well funded or readily available, they represent attempts to fill a void of unmet social and recreational needs that are missing from a current dichotomous treatment model [35].

A Transforming Culture of Recovery

Fortunately, we are in the midst of a transforming culture of recovery in the USA. Recently there has been a push for new recovery support institutions that promote long-standing recovery in the community while maintaining ties to professional treatment for SUD. The response has been the development of a recovery-oriented system. The most prominent example is the Recovery Oriented Community (ROC) which is an independent organization created by and on behalf of people in recovery that promotes advocacy and the creation of recovery resources in communities that have unmet needs [33]. Some of the main strategies of ROCs are to promote recovery education initiations, redesign treatment to reflect the many different pathways to recovery, and enhance the connection between current formal and informal treatment models. Recovery-oriented systems see clinical treatment as an important but singular component to recovery. Instead, these organizations strive to enhance community resources while maintaining links to professional care, enabling a comprehensive approach where recovery can flourish. A prominent theme in this transforming culture is that recovering and recovered people are part of the solution. As such, peers are one of the major strategies employed by recovery support services to increase the prevalence of quality, long-term recovery for those in need [33].

Using Peers to Enhance Access to Treatment

Facilitating Change for Those Not in Treatment

Peers have the potential to help facilitate treatment initiation for individuals who have not yet done so themselves. This is a critical population to engage because the vast majority of people with a substance use disorder do not receive treatment for it (SAMHSA). Epidemiological research has shown that the main reason for this striking statistic has to do with discrepancy in perceived need for treatment. In 2018, 95% of people aged 12 and older with an active, untreated SUD did not perceive any need for treatment. For those who perceived a need for treatment, the most common reason for not receiving it was ambivalence about cessation – two in five did not feel ready to stop using (SAMHSA). Other reasons for not being in treatment despite having a SUD and a perceived need for treatment have to do with stigma related to seeking help and access-related issues, for example, not knowing where to find treatment or not being able to afford the cost [29].

Individuals who do not feel they need treatment or who aren't ready to change represent a challenging and vulnerable population for clinicians to intervene on. The question becomes how to help these individuals if they don't ask for it or even feel they need it? While it may not be to solicit treatment for substance use, these individuals have a high chance of presenting to clinical settings for medical sequelae related to their substance use, making this an opportune time to intervene. Depending on the circumstances, these instances can often be "eye-opening" experiences, and studies have shown that this is a critical time to engage a patient in discussions about use reduction or cessation because they may be more motivated to change their behavior [13].

However, there can be many barriers that get in the way of making a meaningful intervention in this critical time frame. There is significant stigmatization associated with healthcare settings, and fear of judgment may make an individual less likely to want to engage with treatment-related resources even if they are provided to them. Unintentional negative countertransference from the healthcare provider may make the individual with a SUD feel hesitant to disclose information about their substance use or ask for help for it [2]. In addition, the clinical language and the general basis of a clinical relationship – bound by ethical considerations like not forming intimate bonds – can also be a major barrier to capitalizing on these instances. Because peers operate from their own lived experience with both substance use and the struggle of recovery, they may be uniquely poised to make interventions in these settings. Research into the overall impact of peer-based interactions on patients with SUD show that peers bolster the patient's sense of feeling heard and supported [6]. Therefore, peers may represent an important resource that can mitigate some of the stigma that otherwise limits how meaningful these initial interactions can be.

Based on what we know about the stages of change and motivation, it is best to meet individuals where they are rather than force them into a stage of change they may not have arrived at on their own [10]. Therefore, the primary goal of interacting with individuals who are against or on the fence about treatment should be to establish a positive connection, rather than focus on treatment initiation. Because they have been there themselves, peers understand that initiating recovery is riddled with nuances. Peer services in general are rooted in the stages of change, and interactions with peers are dictated by the client's stage of motivation – be it to stop using or just to consider that their substance use may be problematic. Peer-support workers utilize language based on common experience rather than clinical terminology, and can appear more credible than healthcare professionals when it comes to talk about drug use or recovery, and therefore may be more likely to inspire meaningful change [22]. Studies have shown that a consistent result from peer-delivered services across a variety of different settings is that they promote individual self-awareness about problematic substance use. This is important because even if an individual is not ready to change, improved recognition about problematic use increases the likelihood of an individual taking future steps toward initiating recovery [12].

Bernstein et al. showed even a brief peer interaction targeted toward promoting recovery can result in meaningful changes in substance use. This randomized controlled trial took place in a walk-in clinic for individuals presenting with heroin and/or cocaine use in the past 90 days but who were not currently receiving any substance use treatment ($n = 1175$). Both groups received written advice about SUD and a list of referrals for treatment, but the intervention group also spoke with a peer before leaving the clinic who attempted to engage the patient in a conversation about drug cessation and provide a real-life example of what recovery could look like. At 6 months the intervention group was more likely to be abstinent or trending toward abstinence. The findings in this study are encouraging and suggest that peers can meaningfully influence individuals who are on the fence about treatment. More sustained contact might even strengthen the intervention [4].

Peers in Emergency Rooms

A unique opportunity to intervene is in the case of an individual who is in an emergency room after being revived from opioid overdose. These individuals are at high risk for recurrent overdoses and death, so this represents a crucial moment to connect. However, many emergency rooms do not have the appropriate workforce to make this connection, and professionals who are in a position to intervene are limited in their time and experience on the topic. Moreover, emergency room providers are inundated with the most severe cases of SUD and related problems, and emergency room staff may have provided the same resources multiple times to a single patient who continues to use. Consequently, professionals in this setting may have a higher burden of negative countertransference toward this patient population, and this can perpetuate feelings of perceived negative judgment by the patient. It is not uncommon for overdose survivors to leave with limited and generic resources for care, or to leave before any intervention has been made at all [22].

Recently there have been efforts to incorporate peers into emergency room settings. There are a variety of different ways peers can help engage survivors of overdoses in the immediate time frame surrounding the event. Peers can present at the bedside after a patient has been stabilized and before discharge to deliver important information about recovery such as where to find support groups or what types of medications are available for opioid use disorders. Peers do not have to abide by the same constraints as medical professionals and are encouraged to share their own story with the patient. And to a patient who feels hopeless, peers can model that a life in recovery is possible [11].

Another innovative use of peers in the emergency room is for harm reduction strategies. Peers are being trained on how to teach patients about the administration of naloxone in the event of a future overdose. There is a hope that this approach is more effective than when the information is given by a clinician or by written instructions [27]. Peers can also provide education about needle exchange programs for IV drug users and help mitigate the problem of HIV/hepatitis [12]. When delivered by an individual in recovery, this potentially lifesaving information can feel more approachable and palatable. These strategies to help curb the burden of disease contribute to a larger effort to connect with individuals in acute care settings who are not yet in treatment and prevent these instances from becoming missed opportunities.

Peers May Be Able to Facilitate Treatment Initiation and Increase the Provision of Addiction-Related Services in Hard-to-Reach Populations

The numerous risk factors for problematic substance use across different populations are well documented. Many of these high-risk populations are also more likely to fall into the category of individuals who have not been treated or do not seek out help. Studies that look at the impact of peer-based recovery supports on some of these hard-to-reach populations are promising [12]. Peers can be incorporated into a variety of different settings and, because of their broad definition and job description, can creatively intervene in ways professional treaters cannot. Below are some encouraging examples of peer-based services having a positive impact on hard-to-reach populations.

Rural Areas
An individual with a SUD who is living in a rural community faces several unique treatment-related challenges. Prevention and treatment resources may be nonexistent or require the individual to travel long distances to reach. The available medical centers may not be equipped with the resources to help intervene with severe drug use disorders. Additionally, limited treatment resources likely correlate to a lack of education about problematic substance use and a limited understanding about what getting help might mean. Boyd et al. showed that brief peer-counseling interventions to women with HIV in rural areas led to an increase in recognition about problematic alcohol use and initiation of steps being taken to address the problem [7]. Hard-to-reach geographic areas may represent an exciting area to continue studying the

effects of peers, who seem to have the potential to increase educational efforts about problematic substance use and help inspire contemplation about initiating treatment. This may represent a more cost-effective approach than efforts focused toward creating new treatment institutions.

Smaller more rural communities also can be riddled with more privacy issues or negative stigma that makes admitting to a substance use issue demoralizing and initiating steps to change the behavior seem less accessible and desirable. Kelley et al. explored the impact of a community-driven peer-support intervention among a Native American community in Montana. The goals were to increase sobriety but also promote community awareness about substance use problems, which, in turn, can challenge existing stigma in such a community. Involvement in the peer-recovery support program led to decreased substance use and also promoted community-level changes reflected in increased attendance at self-help groups and increased perceived level of support by family and friends.

Other High-Risk Communities

Urban settings are often filled with higher rates of problematic substance use, perhaps because of the various cultural- and societal-level risk factors at play. In these communities, neighborhood poverty and violence increase vulnerability to drug use. Drug use may also be deeply entwined with the family and peer groups of a given individual. Laws that protect communities from illegal selling of drugs may be less strict, meaning there is easier access to illegal drugs (SAMHSA). These risk factors are often negatively correlated with seeking help and initiating treatment and represent another domain where peers may be particularly useful in engaging at-risk individuals.

Deering et al. studied a unique peer-led intervention among a sample of female sex workers working in an urban setting. Drug use is common in this line of work, and those employed in the sex industry are particularly high-risk for developing SUD in addition to being at risk for sexually transmitted infections and violence. The study examined the impact of a peer-led mobile outreach program to examine whether it was correlated with increased use of addiction treatment services. The program was in place for over 18 months, and at the end, findings showed that women who used the program were more likely to subsequently enter inpatient addiction treatment including detoxification and rehabilitation. The higher-risk women (those employed in more isolated settings and with higher client volume) were actually the most likely to utilize the peer-run service, suggesting that peers may be critical for engaging a population that would otherwise fall through the cracks.

In another outreach study, peers approached people off the street in identified areas for high-risk opioid use and overdose. Peers were instructed to engage individuals in a conversation about heroin and then offer the individual involvement in a study to help initiate treatment for OUD. If interested, the peer then directly facilitated entry into the study by calling clinical staff and initiating a phone screen. If eligible, the participant was brought to the study site where they met with a professional who would link them to either detoxification or methadone agonist medication therapy (MAT). Almost 100% of the individuals that were identified and deemed eligible for the study actually showed up to the treatment linkage meeting and subsequently became engaged in either detoxification or were admitted for MAT. Follow-up studies showed that the majority of these individuals remained in treatment even after 60 days. While there was no comparison group to see how non-peer providers might fare in connecting individuals to linkage appointments, peers seemed to have an overwhelming success rate in facilitating treatment for a population that professionals may have limited success in engaging. This highlights an exciting synergistic potential use of peers into the framework of professionally delivered care.

Using Peers to Improve Treatment Engagement

Treatment Retention

Once in treatment, a significant challenge becomes how to keep people in treatment until completion. Poor treatment retention has been a long-standing problem that interferes with treatment success [13]. In the report from last year, the Substance Abuse and Mental Health Services Administration (SAMHSA) found that almost 60% of clients leave formal substance use treatment prior to completion, regardless of the treatment setting or the type of substance used.

Studies have shown that when compared to traditional treatment alone, individuals who have some type of peer-support intervention are more likely to complete programs for SUD. Blondell et al. studied peer-counseling interventions in a detoxification unit and found that individuals who received even a single peer-counseling session were more likely than those who did not to complete medical detoxification and not leave against medical advice. Moreover, those individuals with a peer intervention were more likely to attend already available 12-Step meetings offered as part of the hospitalization and were more likely to initiate aftercare [5]. It is not uncommon for detox units to have 12-Step groups available, but the extent to which patients engage with these is variable. This study and others similar to it suggest that there is some unique, added benefit of a one-on-one peer intervention where the peer was able to share their own recovery experience and encourage a meaningful connection to already available mutual aid modalities [18].

A vexing problem for providers is that many patients who complete detox do not follow up with appropriate aftercare resources. This is a recipe for relapse and poor outcomes. As mentioned above, Blondell showed that individuals who interacted with peers while hospitalized for detox also were more likely to follow up with professional SUD aftercare, suggesting that peer interventions in structured inpatient settings may translate to better engagement with outpatient care [5]. Similarly, work by Tracy et al. showed that peer-support interventions delivered to a group of veterans who were hospitalized on inpatient units led to enhanced post-discharge aftercare adherence ($n = 96$). Peer interventions included weekly peer mentorship and peer-led relapse prevention groups and were compared to treatment as usual (which in addition to clinical care included supports in the form of coping skills groups and standard social work support). Peer interventions were superior to treatment as usual (which was not devoid of personalized support), suggesting something unique in the interaction between patients and peers that may promote better adherence. Peers may inspire feelings of competency and agency over their substance use disorder in ways that non-peers cannot. In addition, the increased adherence transcended to general medical aftercare as well, further supporting this idea [31].

The value of mutual aid modalities in supporting long-standing recovery has already been discussed, as has the fact that physicians can play a role in promoting these programs but that this intervention is prone to falling short. Manning et al. examined whether peer referral to 12-Step meetings increased meeting attendance among individuals on an inpatient detox unit compared to those who were referred by a doctor or had no referral at all but had access to the meetings. The results showed that peer introduction and referral to 12-Step programs by both peers and doctors increased meeting attendance while inpatient and after discharge and that post-discharge attendance was highest in the peer referral group. The individuals who attended meetings post-discharge trended toward higher abstinence rates [18]. This is another way that peers can bridge the gap between professional and informal care.

Peers Help Improve the Relationship to Treatment and Treatment Providers

Studies have shown that structured treatment for SUD works best when individuals feel positively about the treatment – be it through the relationships with treatment providers or through the provision of care. Studies have shown that one of the best predictors for successful treatment outcomes has to do with engagement, which Yang et al. define as "treatment participation and positive treatment experience" [39]. Those providing and receiving care are essential to the process of treatment engagement, but clinicians often see barriers to treatment as a client-driven issue (i.e., poor motivation), whereas clients are more likely to feel less engaged because of the environment and staff. Yang et al. used a qualitative approach and interviewed patients in an inpatient substance use treatment program to investigate factors that impacted treatment engagement and found that the therapeutic relationship with the treatment provider is an essential component to feeling satisfied with treatment overall. As already mentioned, peers have a unique ability to connect on a therapeutic level due to the process of mutuality. They may be able to play an important role with helping patients feel more supported in treatment and improving individuals' relationships with their existing treatment providers [39].

Sanders et al. examined the impact of peer-driven relationships for women already involved in a program to address their SUD. Women who received ongoing counseling from a peer found this intervention to be one of the most helpful aspects of the program overall. Peers were described as empathetic and were able to establish greater rapport with the patient compared to the clinic professionals. While the study does not speak to overall treatment outcomes regarding substance use, the women who received support from a peer counselor were more likely to recommend the treatment to others and more likely to utilize the available resources already available through the clinic [28].

Andreas et al. examined the impact of incorporating peers into the framework of a substance use recovery program for individuals with SUD and history of incarceration. Peers were women into the approach to treatment through groups, coaching, and workshops and also facilitated community-level support by providing links to sober recreational activities and community events. Authors of the study found that individuals engaged in this program had increases in self-efficacy and perception of social support and quality of life [1]. This is promising work because individuals with criminal justice backgrounds are especially vulnerable to relapse. Peers have the potential to mitigate this risk by enhancing positive feelings about treatment which in turn promotes treatment effectiveness in a population where treatment is otherwise associated with poor outcomes.

Using Peers to Promote Enduring Recovery

Treatment represents only a short time in the context of lifelong recovery. Perhaps one of the most daunting tasks is maintaining recovery once it has been achieved. While reduction in substance use is often necessary to initiate recovery, there are a variety of separate challenges that have the potential to interfere with the process of achieving enduring recovery. Without sufficient recovery capital – a term used to describe the internal and external resources that can be drawn upon to help sustain recovery – a newly recovered individual is vulnerable to poor outcomes [38]. Peers become distinctly useful in the context of promoting recovery capital and helping an individual succeed in their plan for reducing or eliminating substances long-term. The peer relationship is often heavily focused on providing a newly recovered individual with tools, resources, and support, and peers can help create recovery plans customized to meet an individual's recovery needs and goals [29].

The Many Benefits of Improved Social Support on Recovery

The likelihood of relapse rises if a person is lacking in personal and social support, representing an opportune area for peer intervention [21]. In fact, one of the most consistent benefits of peer support, regardless of the setting and context in which they are utilized, is an increase in social support and perception of community affiliation [6]. A primary role of peer-support interventions is to ensure that those in early recovery are hooked up to support networks with social resources. They help an individual construct their own recovery-oriented network which can be made up of various mutual aid groups and social or community programs, all of which provide healthy, sober contexts for a person newly in recovery to find support. It also seems that the presence of a social network can impact how meaningfully an individual engages with ongoing treatment. One study looked at the impact of a peer-led social group on individuals with co-occurring mental illness and SUD who were recently discharged from the hospital. Those who were involved in the social group had higher levels of outpatient service use in the short term, and decreased substance use in the long term [24]. Similarly, Andreas et al. looked at the effects of the Peers Reach Out Supporting Peers to Embrace Recovery (PROSPER) program which is a recovery community run by peers who are focused on individuals with substance use who are reentering society from the prison system. In this program, peers were paid a stipend; were formally trained and supervised by program staff to lead groups, workshops, and seminars; and directly linked individuals to recreational activities and social and community events. From baseline to 12-month assessment, there were observable increases in self-efficacy, social support, and quality of life [1]. While not directly related to substance use outcomes, it is reasonable to assume that these factors which relate to self-esteem and confidence can improve one's ability to feel equipped to manage a life in recovery. Follow-up studies on PROSPER using the Government Performance and Results Act datasets found that housing stability nearly tripled and probation/parole status decreased from 82% to 32% [3]. These results support the idea that peer-based services intervene in ways that traditional treatment approaches do not but that this approach is particularly useful for individuals with limited recovery capital, such as those with a history of incarceration and a high risk for relapse without sufficient concrete support like stable housing.

Peers Improving Outpatient Treatment Adherence

Outpatient treatment programs can be an important part of long-standing recovery, but insufficient recovery capital can limit how well someone can engage with this treatment. Laudet et al. investigated retention issues in an outpatient substance use treatment setting and determined three major factors responsible for early dropout: clients felt that the treatment program did not have supportive staff, lacked in provision of social services (e.g., job training, help with housing, childcare, stable housing), and did not provide enough flexibility to accommodate external responsibilities [16]. These deficits in recovery resources lead to an individual feeling ill-equipped to meet the demands of early recovery. This represents a major structural flaw in current treatment which often neglects the challenges that can threaten a life in recovery. Peer services are often directly targeted to fill this gap and not only promote engagement with outpatient treatment, but lay the framework for long-standing recovery in individuals who are vulnerable to relapse.

Tracy and Burton et al. looked at the impact of inpatient peer mentorship services on post-discharge treatment attendance in a VA inpatient cohort ($n = 96$) with substance use and a history of high recidivism. The peer intervention was titled mentorship for alcohol problems (MAP) and included peer-support groups and individual mentorship for alcohol use disorders. Three groups were compared: (1) treatment as usual (TAU) with (2) TAU combined with enhanced dual recovery treatment and MAP (3) dual recovery treatment with MAP. The peers in this case were paid and participated for a total of 6 months. In terms of post-discharge adherence, the two groups which included a peer intervention had higher discharge adherence rates of 43% (Group 2) and 48% (Group 3) compared to 33% in the TAU group [31].

Similarly, Mangrum et al. looked at a peer-inspired program called Access to Recovery (ATR) and how this nontraditional intervention which consisted of direct recovery and social support might improve substance use and substance use-related outcomes in a criminal justice population with significant substance use. This population was referred from drug courts, probation, or child protective services and was not necessarily seeking out treatment on their own. Treatment as usual (without access to recovery substance use supports) was compared to an experimental group who received an ATR which allowed them to access many peer-led recovery services. These included individualized recovery coaching, recovery support groups, relapse prevention groups, and spiritual support groups. According to self-reported data and data from the provider system, those who actually completed their required treatment were significantly more likely to have received the peer-recovery support groups. Better substance use outcomes were also associated with those who had drug court or probation as part of their follow-up. This suggests that peer interventions could synergistically improve compliance with mandated treatments and inspire hope for this population who might not feel recovery is attainable given the traditional lack of support in standard treatment options [17].

Reduced Relapse Rates

Min et al. retrospectively assessed the impact of long-term peer interventions on individuals with mental illness and SUD. They found that the individuals engaged in peer-support programs stayed out of the hospital longer and had lower overall rehospitalizations [20]. Those with co-occurring mental illness and SUD are a challenging population to treat. They represent a significant portion of all inpatient stays and often have longer stays than someone with only one diagnosis [25]. This population tends to be rehospitalized often, and it can be assumed that these individuals have difficulty time functioning in the community. Peer services seem to be an important resource for helping mitigate this issue. This is an example of peer-based services providing unique longitudinal support for individuals who otherwise have significant struggles existing in the community while staying sober. Boisevert et al. showed that a population with co-occurring mental illness and substance use living in supportive permanent housing who were offered a peer-driven recovery program (based on SAMHSA model) were less likely to relapse to substance use compared to residents who did not engage with peer work. The benefits extended beyond sobriety; those involved in the peer-based intervention had lower rates of return to homelessness [6]. Those who participated in the peer program reported increased emotional and informational support which are two of the major support mechanisms of all peer-support services (see Table 1.2). While this was a small population (only ten individuals participated in the peer program), it is an encouraging outcome that suggests additional peer-driven services may enhance the benefits provided by supportive housing and other interventions designed to help high-risk individuals prone to relapse and homelessness by nature of their dual diagnoses and poor recovery capital.

Decreased Criminal Justice Involvement

In a randomized controlled trial, Rowe et al. compared an experimental intervention of group and peer support (in addition to clinical care) to standardized clinical treatment alone in a group of 114 individuals with criminal justice histories, substance use, and mental illness. The peer mentors all had personal history of mental illness and either a history of drug or alcohol use disorders or criminal justice backgrounds. In this study peer mentors were paid staff, and they met with study participants in a one-on-one setting each month. In addition to focusing on sobriety and reduction of substance use, peers emphasized the importance of personal goal setting and development of coping skills and taught participants how to advocate for services. Those in the experimental group who received peer-based interventions had significantly lower levels of drug and alcohol use at both 6 and 12 months of follow-up compared to the control group, who actually increased in the amount of alcohol they used. A secondary outcome was that criminal justice charges decreased significantly for both groups [26]. While the effect size was relatively small, results suggest that peer supports can be a promising adjunct to clinically delivered care for hard-to-treat populations.

Peers to Help Those Already in Long-Standing Recovery

Those already in sustained recovery can also benefit meaningfully from peer-based recovery services. Collegiate recovery programs are growing in availability as a support option for people in recovery in academic settings. Laudet et al. looked into university students who were participating in peer-based college recovery support programs. The study survey identified 486 college students who were abstinent from substances for a mean of 3 years and engaged in various existing college recovery programs. Those in the survey seemed to credit the peer-based programs as tremendously supportive; one third of the sample said they would not be in college if not for their respective peer program. Many individuals believed that without a peer program, their ability to actually succeed in college would be threatened [15]. Peer-recovery programs seem to be important resources for individuals who would otherwise potentially feel alienated or severely challenged by the traditional social environment on college campuses. Other community-based peer programs have been associated with sustained recovery for that particular population, and many outcomes of peer interventions suggest that being the peer delivering recovery advice can be meaningful for one's own recovery maintenance (Armitage). This is similar to the benefits that are conferred by being a sponsor in 12-Step where being in the position of providing support can bolster one's own security in their status as a recovered person [30].

Limitations

While the available body of research suggests that the incorporation of peers in recovery interventions has a positive impact on substance use outcomes, it is important to acknowledge the many limitations in studying this newly developing field. Peers are being used across a variety of different settings and populations and intervene in a myriad of unique ways. They can be paid service professionals or volunteers. This flexibility is useful in terms of real-world applicability, but from a research perspective, it makes for many challenges. There are many methodological issues that limit the ability to draw definitive conclusions about the effectiveness of peer-related interventions [3].

Currently there is no single definition for peer-recovery support services and no standardized training program or manual. Many of the studies referenced in this chapter had varying or poorly defined peer roles, and there was no universal manual for peer certification or provision of treatment, making it challenging to draw upon best practice for specific peer interventions. In response to the rising advocacy and funding for substance use and related programs, we are seeing the creation of various formal integration plans for peer-recovery support services. For example, peer services are now considered a vital component to the way New York State is addressing the opioid epidemic, and there is a push to integrate peers into applicable clinical settings by way of a formal certification and training process [23].

As the culture of recovery continues to change and peers become more recognized as part of the solution, there will be a need for clear cost benefit research which will no doubt expand the knowledge base for utilizing peer-based recovery supports in general. Until then, there continues to be a need for robust studies that closely examine the amount, intensity, skill level, and training profile for which peers should be utilized in order to have the greatest benefit. For example, there is a paucity of large randomized controlled trials with credible comparison treatments in the available body of research. In addition, many of these studies utilize peers across a wide variety of settings and using differing levels of support and interventions, making it hard to parse out the benefits that are unique to what type of peer-led intervention. Research where peers intervene on inpatient units shows that brief interventions like this can be cost-effective ways to boost adherence and engagement [5, 4]. But there is also a need to closely examine additional service contexts for which peer interventions can be of value with differentiation between outpatient, residential, transitional care settings and recovery community settings. These clinical populations may differ in their needs and this would consequently impact the ways peers are applied.

Conclusion

This chapter highlights the various ways peer-support recovery services can enhance the current approach to treating SUD. Professionally delivered treatments can be useful for intervening on the acute recovery needs like assisting with cessation or addressing life-threatening issues, but there are gaps in this approach because many individuals do not successfully complete treatment, feel connected or helped by treatment, or feel that treatment is easily accessible. Some of this void has organically been filled by mutual aid programs – mostly 12-Step– which has its own well-articulated use of peer supports, but these groups are only a singular pathway to long-standing recovery and also do not fit the needs of each individual patient with a unique recovery journey. Many clinical professionals feel that peer treatment is equivalent to 12-Step, but this chapter shows how there are numerous other ways in which peers can be incorporated into the existing framework for substance use treatment. However, peers are currently under-applied and under-recognized in terms of their potential applications. Existing literature shows the potential of peer-based support interventions across many different settings where struggling individuals with undertreated SUD exist. Peers have a promising place in this area of recovery; the existing body of literature suggests that peer-recovery services have the potential to make it easier for people to find and connect meaningfully to existing treatment. Moreover, peer-support interventions target the process of helping newly recovered individuals plan and rebuild a life that can withstand the many challenges that interfere with enduring recovery.

As the culture of recovery changes, there is room for peer work to grow and improve. Nonstructured peer-style interventions are rising in popularity as evidenced by social savvy media platforms promoting sober-curiosity movements. There is no doubt that the impact of personalized stories, devoid of stigma, is tremendously powerful on an individual who is struggling with problematic substance use. But without more robust research into the effective incorporation of peers into existing SUD treatment, we run the risk of letting the pace be set by wellness leaders and social influencers who are not professionally trained or necessarily have the best interests of patients in mind. Currently we have not sorted out the optimal way to apply peer interventions in the numerous pathways to recovery, but peer interventions across a variety of different settings and contexts intervene in valuable ways that professional treatment does not traditionally address. Limitations with studying peer work are nontrivial and need to be considered in the years to come; however, the general conclusion is that peer-based recovery support services represent an exciting new intervention in the field of recovery.

References

1. Andreas D, Ja DY, Wilson S. Peers reach out supporting peers to embrace recovery (PROSPER): a center for substance abuse treatment recovery community services program. Alcohol Treat Q. 2010;28(3):326–38.
2. Avery J. The stigma of addiction in the medical community. An Essential Guide. 2019. https://doi.org/10.1007/978-3-030-02580-9_6.
3. Bassuk E, Hanson J, Greene N, et al. Peer delivered recovery support services for addictions in the United States: a systematic review. J Subst Abus Treat. 2016;63:1–9.
4. Bernstein J, Bernstein E, Tassiopoulos K, et al. Brief motivational intervention at a clinic visit reduces cocaine and heroin use. Drug Alcohol Depend. 2005;77:49–59.
5. Blondell RD, Behrens T, Smith S, et al. Peer support during inpatient detoxification and aftercare outcomes. Addict Dis Their Treat. 2008;7:77–86.
6. Boisvert RA, Martin LM, Grosek M, et al. Effectiveness of a peer-support community in addiction recovery: participation as intervention. Occup Ther Int. 2008;15(4):205–20.
7. Boyd MR, Moneyham L, Murdaugh C, et al. A peer-based substance abuse intervention for HIV+ rural women: A pilot study. Archives of Psychiatric Nursing. 2005;19(1):10–7.
8. Center for Substance Abuse Treatment. What are peer recovery support services? HHS publication no. (SMA) 09-4454. Rockville: Substance Abuse and Mental Health Services Administration, U.S. Department of Health and Human Services; 2009.
9. Center for Substance Abuse Treatment. An introduction to mutual support groups for alcohol and drug abuse, Substance abuse in brief fact sheet, vol. 5, Issue 1. Rockville: Substance Abuse and Mental Health Services Administration; 2008.
10. DiClemente CC, Schlundt D, Gemmell L. Readiness and stages of change in addiction treatment. Am J Addict. 2004;13:103–19.
11. D'Onofrio G, O'Connor PG, Pantalon MV, et al. Emergency department–initiated buprenorphine/naloxone treatment for opioid dependence: a randomized clinical trial. JAMA. 2015;313(16):1636–44.
12. Eddie D, Hoffman L, Vilsaint C, et al. Lived experience in new models of care for substance use disorder: a systematic review of peer recovery support services and recovery coaching. Front Psychol. 2019;10:2–12.
13. Fiorentine R, Nakashima J, Anglin MD. Client engagement in drug treatment. J Subst Abus Treat. 1997;17:199–206.

14. Humphreys K. Circles of recovery: self-help organizations for addictions. London: Cambridge University Press; 2004.
15. Laudet AB, Harris K, Kimball T, et al. In college and in recovery: reasons for joining a collegiate recovery program. J Am Coll Heal. 2016;64:238–46.
16. Laudet AB, Humphreys K. Promoting recovery in an evolving policy context: what do we know and what do we need to know about recovery support services? J Subst Abus Treat. 2013;45(1):126–33.
17. Mangrum L. Final evaluation report: creating access to recovery through drug courts. Austin, Texas Department of State Health Services. Mental Health and Substance Abuse Services Division. Gulf Coast Addiction Technology Transfer Center: Austin; 2008.
18. Manning V, Best D, Faulkner N, et al. Does active referral by a doctor or 12-step peer improve 12-step meeting attendance? Results from a pilot randomised control trial. Drug Alcohol Dep. 2012;126:131–7.
19. McCrady B, Tonigan JS. Chapter 68: Recent research into twelve step programs. In: Ries RK, Fiellin DA, Miller SC, Saitz R, editors. Principles of addiction medicine. 4th edn. Philadelphia, PA: Lippincott Williams & Wilkins; 2009.
20. Min SY, Whitecraft E, Rothbard AB, Salzer MS. Peer support for persons with co-occurring disorders and community tenure: A survival analysis. Psychiatric Rehabilitation Journal. 2007;30(3):207–13.
21. Moos RH, Moos BS. Rates and predictors of relapse after natural and treated remission from alcohol use disorders. Addiction. 2006;101(2):212–22.
22. National Council for Behavioral Health. Peer support workers in emergency departments: engaging individuals surviving opioid overdoses–qualitative assessment. Retrieved from: https://www.thenationalcouncil.org/wp-content/uploads/2018/12/Peer-Support-Workers-in-EDs-Issue-Brief.pdf.
23. New York State Office of Alcoholism and Substance Abuse Services. Peer integration and the stages of change toolKit. 2018. Retrieved from: https://oasas.ny.gov/system/files/documents/2019/08/PeerIntegrationToolKit-DigitalFinal.pdf.
24. O'Connell MJ, Flanagan E, Delphin M, et al. Enhancing outcomes for persons with co-occurring disorders through skills training and peer recovery support. J Ment Health. 2017;10:1–6.
25. Owens PL, Fingar KR, McDermott KW, et al. Inpatient stays involving mental and substance use disorders, 2016. HCUP statistical brief #249. March 2019. Agency for Healthcare Research and Quality, Rockville. www.hcup-us.ahrq.gov/reports/statbriefs/sb249-Mental-Substance-Use-Disorder-Hospital-Stays-2016.pdf.
26. Rowe M, Bellamy C, Baranoski M, et al. A peer-support, group intervention to reduce substance use and criminality among persons with severe mental illness. Psychiatric Services. 2007;58(7):955–61.

27. Samuels EA, Bernstein SL, Marshall BDL, et al. Peer navigation and take-home naloxone for opioid overdose emergency department patients: preliminary patient outcomes. J Subst Abus Treat. 2018;94:29–34.
28. Sanders L, Trinh C, Sherman B, et al. Assessment of client satisfaction in a peer counseling substance abuse treatment program for pregnant and postpartum women. Eval Program Plann. 1998;21:287–96.
29. Substance Abuse and Mental Health Services Administration Office of Applied Studies Treatment Episode Data Set (TEDS) 2005. Discharges from substance abuse treatment services, DASIS Series. Rockville: Substance Abuse and Mental Health Services Administration; 2017.
30. Schulz JE, Williams V, Galligan JE. Chapter 67: Twelve step programs in recovery. In: Ries RK, Fiellin DA, Miller SC, Saitz R, editors. Principles of addiction medicine. 4th edn. Philadelphia, PA: Lippincott Williams & Wilkins; 2009.
31. Tracy K, Burton M, Nich C, et al. Utilizing peer mentorship to engage high recidivism substance-abusing patients in treatment. Am J Drug Alcohol Abuse. 2011;37(6):525–31.
32. Tracy K, Wallace SP. Benefits of peer support groups in the treatment of addiction. Subst Abus Rehabil. 2016;7:143–54.
33. Valentine P, White W, Taylor P. The recovery community organization: toward a definition. 2007. Posted at http://www.facesandvoicesofrecovery.org/pdf/valentine_white_taylor_2007.pdf.
34. Williams A. The New Sobriety. New York Times [Internet]. 2019 June 15; Style. Available from: https://www.nytimes.com/2019/06/15/style/sober-curious.html.
35. White WL, Kelly JF, Roth JD. New addiction-recovery support institutions: mobilizing support beyond professional addiction treatment and recovery mutual aid. J Groups Addict Recov. 2012;7:297–31.
36. White W, Kurtz E. The varieties of recovery experience. Int J Self Help Self Care. 2006;3(1–2):21–61.
37. White WL, Evans AC. The recovery agenda: the shared role of peers and professionals. Public Health Rev. 2014;35(2):1–15.
38. White W, Cloud W. Recovery capital: a primer for addictions professionals. Counselor. 2008;9(5):22–7.
39. Yang Y, Perkins D, Stearns A. Barriers and facilitators to treatment engagement among clients in inpatient substance abuse treatment. Qual Health Res. 2018;28(9):1474–85.

Peer Support for Mental Health

2

Ana Stefancic, Lauren Bochicchio, and Daniela Tuda

Introduction

Peer Support for Mental Health

One in four people (approximately 450 million people worldwide) has a diagnosable mental health condition, making mental illness one of the leading causes of disability [47]. Mental illness can significantly impair quality of life and make it difficult to sustain employment, stable housing, and relationships and to engage in activities of daily living. The burden of mental illness is also associated with increased rates of certain physical health conditions, such as cardiovascular disease, and premature mortality, particularly for those diagnosed with conditions such as schizophrenia or bipolar disorder [21, 46]. Given the widespread prevalence and impact of mental illness, it is critical to understand and disseminate supports that can enhance quality of life and mental health recovery.

A. Stefancic (✉) · D. Tuda
Columbia University, Department of Psychiatry, New York, NY, USA
e-mail: as2463@columbia.edu; dt2537@columbia.edu

L. Bochicchio
Columbia University School of Nursing, New York, NY, USA
e-mail: lab2223@cumc.columbia.edu

Within mental health, the term peer refers to an individual who self-identifies as having a mental illness and/or as a current or former user of mental health services who draws upon their personal experience to support others, either formally or informally. Depending on the context, personal experience may be coupled with specialized training in service delivery. By tapping into their lived experience and often knowledge or skills gained from training, peers help promote wellness and recovery among others facing similar challenges [43].

Though peer support within mental health has an extensive history, its modern roots are in the peer/consumer/survivor/recovery advocacy movements, as well as the broader disability and civil rights movements, that sought (and still seek) to drastically shift the processes and outcomes of care for people with mental illness. Advocates aimed to disrupt traditional mental health treatment that often isolated, stigmatized, mistreated, and denied the autonomy and personhood of people with mental illness. Advocates further sought to move beyond an emphasis on symptom reduction as the objective of mental healthcare toward the promotion of broader recovery, social inclusion, and quality of life as key goals and processes. Altogether, emphasis would be placed on individualized journeys for people to "improve their health and wellness, live self-directed lives, and strive to reach their full potential" [42]. By building peer networks, coalitions, and communities, new supports arose that would respect personhood, foster hope, and empower individuals with mental illness [35].

Peer support for mental health is characterized by self-disclosure and sharing of experiences of mental illness, treatment, and other challenges, as well as strategies and successes, in efforts to reduce isolation, combat stigma, and promote hope, empowerment, and recovery. Most commonly, modalities of peer support for mental health can be categorized as participation in mutual support, peer-run organizations, and peer-delivered services (also known as peer support services). Mutual support consists of both one-on-one and group support that is generally characterized by a more informal nature, high levels of reciprocity, and participation of individuals who are not paid professional service providers [19]. Similarly, peer-run organizations are usually distinguished by having a majority of their staff, leadership, and governing bodies (e.g., board of directors) comprised of individuals who self-identify as peers [32]. These organizations generally offer a combination of informal and mutual peer support, more formal peer-delivered services, as well as peer engagement in social action and advocacy. Finally, peer-delivered services also offer both one-on-one and group support but are generally more formal, characterized by lower reciprocity, and often involve paid peer providers [22]. Peer providers are often embedded within mainstream mental health agencies, and while they often acknowledge and appreciate the possibility of learning from or feeling supported by the individuals they serve, this is not an expectation that is placed on the service users.

In the following sections, we provide in-depth descriptions of the types of peer support available for mental health, how they are thought to work, and the research regarding their effectiveness. We focus additional attention on peer-delivered services, as they represent one of the most rapidly growing and studied areas of peer support, discussing both challenges and opportunities encountered by the peer workforce in mental health. Throughout, we offer quotes from qualitative research that provide an opportunity for peer voices to be heard. Finally, we offer strategies for further expanding the reach and impact of peer support, along with recommendations for future research.

Types of Peer-Based Support in Mental Health

Mutual Peer Support

In its broadest sense, mutual support for mental health can be defined as the affiliation of people who share similar mental health difficulties and interact regularly to exchange information and give and receive support [33]. Sometimes referred to as mutual aid or self-help, mutual support ranges from formally organized mutual support groups (e.g., Beating Bipolar, Recovery International, Schizophrenics Anonymous, GROW) to highly informal one-to-one exchanges. It generally offers access to nonprofessional, unpaid networks where peers can identify with one another, share experiences of challenges and resilience, and benefit by virtue of both giving and receiving support. Mutual support often emphasizes social affiliation and fellowship along with an exchange of information (e.g., how to cope with symptoms) and emotional support (e.g., expressing care for one's peers).

Mutual support groups may have a designated leader or facilitator who may be further along in mental health recovery, may have received training, and can serve as a role model, or they may have a nonhierarchical structure with all peers participating equally. Some mutual support groups follow general processes that have been adapted from 12-step programs for alcohol use (e.g., Double Trouble in Recovery), while others offer a less standardized and unstructured approach. Similarly, some mutual support utilizes tools such as Wellness Recovery Action Planning (WRAP) [34] to facilitate peers' exploring their personal recovery, identifying potential stressors, and developing individualized strategies for self-managing their mental health conditions.

Peer-Run Organizations

Peer-run organizations were founded to create communities wherein persons with mental illness could access social affiliation, exercise autonomy and self-direction, give and receive support, and contribute to the operation and functioning of the organization. These organizations cultivate a shared sense of ownership, with emphasis on egalitarianism, flexible organizational structures that encourage member input, voluntary membership/participation, and activities that are facilitated by members. Organizations tend to use both volunteers and paid staff to help operate programs and provide support.

While self-care and mutual support groups are the core supports offered by most peer-run organizations, informal social activities (e.g., lunches, game nights) and peer-delivered support services are also common. Individuals may participate in a mutual support group (e.g., Hearing Voices) or meet individually with a peer provider to discuss financial challenges [32]. Additionally, these organizations provide platforms for peers to engage in advocacy to challenge stigma and discrimination, educate others, and participate in mental health policymaking and planning. Peers may meet with agency leadership to inform internal policies or protocols or participate in an advocacy campaign to increase affordable housing for persons with mental illness.

Peer-Delivered Services

Peer-delivered services have rapidly expanded over the past 20 years, evolving into a workforce of over 30,000 providers in the United States [29]. Peer providers combine their lived experience of mental illness, service use, and formal training to support others. Peer providers may be employed in a variety of settings, but are commonly embedded within mainstream mental health services, or other community-based health and wellness settings (Table 2.1), working alongside non-peer providers [16, 31]. While tasks and responsibilities differ across settings, peer providers generally build rapport with service users, instill hope for change, support self-determination, and help others identify and work toward personal goals. Peer/service user interactions may be highly unstructured or may revolve around structured activities or evidence-based intervention, such as WRAP or Wellness-Self Management [10, 28]. As peer-delivered services have gained traction, roles have been developed as part of services for specific groups of individuals experiencing mental health issues (e.g., youth or older adult peer specialists). Recent efforts have also adapted peer-delivered services beyond mental health, in particular to include aspects of physical health, where peer providers' experience with both mental illness and physical health challenges is essential [2, 5].

Peer providers can also educate their non-peer colleagues and inform mental health service delivery by sharing their perspective. Peer providers are highly focused on aspects of the process of care (e.g., the degree to which provider practice aligns with service users' preferences and needs and promotes autonomy and

Table 2.1 Settings and focus of peer-delivered services

Setting/program type	Sample role of peer provider
Warmlines	Provide nonemergency telephone or virtual support to individuals experiencing mental health challenges, provide information and referrals to community resources based on the callers' needs
Psychiatric emergency department	Provide trauma-informed support to individuals in psychiatric emergency departments by helping them navigate highly stressful processes, advocate for patient rights, and follow up after discharge
Crisis intervention teams	Work in the community with a multidisciplinary team (e.g., psychiatrist, nurse) to prevent or reduce behavioral health crises and support service users' safety in potential encounters with law enforcement
Respite programs	Provide short-term supports in a homelike environment as an alternative to hospitalization or to prevent crisis
Assertive community treatment teams	Provide long-term support to individuals with SMI through outreach and engagement in the community as part of a multidisciplinary team. Support service users with wellness planning, community integration, and recovery goals
Criminal justice/criminal justice diversion	Serve as mentors for individuals navigating the criminal justice system while providing support with the court system and reentry into the community
Hospital Bridger programs	Support individuals transitioning from inpatient care to community living and outpatient care by engaging them in the hospital, assisting with access to community resources, and supporting them with community integration
Employment programs	Support participants with reintegrating into the workforce helping them identify employment-related concerns and strategies. Serve as role models demonstrating the benefits and feasibility of working
Health and wellness	Provide coaching to support wellness, self-management of health conditions, and healthy lifestyles. Collaborate with other community services and assist people to access and navigate healthcare systems
Supportive housing	Provide long-term supports to assist individuals with obtaining and maintaining housing, community integration, and recovery goals

self-determination) and can thus help transform mainstream clinician-directed and outcome-focused care toward more recovery-oriented care. Further, they can also engage in advocacy on behalf of service users, ensuring that their voices are heard and respected both within their organizations and broader systems.

How Does Peer Support Work Within Mental Health?

Peer Approach: "[a peer] takes the time to be patient, understanding, *listen*, point a finger in the right direction"

Regardless of the modality of peer support, its foundation rests on personal experience, perspective, and knowledge of mental health, treatment, and recovery. The language that peers use is generally lay language, rather than clinical, rooted in common experience, and emphasizes strengths rather than deficits. Other essential aspects include a nonlinear view of mental health recovery, the normalization of challenges, and building fulfilling and meaningful lives despite potential ongoing mental health difficulties [22]. Peers acknowledge setbacks occur and validate these experiences as part of the recovery journey, offering opportunities for continued learning and growth rather than being signs of failure [45]. Peers can help others to understand the broader context of these events within their lives, to emphasize the skills that got them through previous challenges, help develop additional ways of coping, and remind them that "tomorrow is a new day." Peers' overall approach involves active listening, disclosure of their own experiences, a nonjudgmental stance toward the experiences of others, and reminding others of their strength and resilience. As one peer describes:

> by talking through what they're going through, all of a sudden it comes as like a light bulb...there's another option that they can think about...that's uh- giving hope, and you can see the hope is still there.

Peers convey empathy and support others with developing coping strategies and skills (e.g., mindfulness activities, engaging supportive networks), problem-solving, and fostering empowerment and self-management of mental health conditions and stressors (e.g., techniques for advocating with clinical treatment providers) [18]. Peer support also offers opportunities for social support and affiliation, which is especially critical for persons with serious mental illness who often experience extreme forms of marginalization and social isolation [45]. In addition, peers often function as role models for individuals in the process of recovery, bolstering hope and empowerment [39].

Traditional mental health services have often imposed clinician-driven goals and dampened people's belief in their capacity to build a meaningful life and pursue goals and dreams. Peer support can help rekindle self-identified goals such as furthering education, obtaining employment, having supportive social networks, developing hobbies, and establishing greater self-sufficiency. Peers can also facilitate access to resources (e.g., housing supports) and other nonprofessional (e.g., AA meetings) or professional mental health services, while also providing support for navigating those services. Finally, all peer interactions should be characterized by openness to diversity, individualized recovery journeys, and cultural humility [4]. Overall, this type of approach challenges stigma and elicits self-acceptance, validation, hope, empowerment, self-efficacy, and a sense of belonging [4].

Shared Experience in Peer-Delivered Services

Much of the success of peer support is attributed to "shared experience," which refers to the background, perspective, and experiences to which peers may relate or have in common. Peers' use of self-disclosure can enhance views of peers as credible sources of support and potential role models; in the words of one participant in peer support services, "you have to make me a believer and you got to tell me *how* you know…You just can't sit there and talk. Not unless you walking the walk." Such disclosure helps others feel more comfortable, facilitates openness, improves hopefulness about the possibility of change, and inspires individuals to take steps toward their own wellness and recovery [2, 39]. For peer providers, their lived experience serves as a "lens" through which they view and understand others' challenges [40]. It shapes their approach to supporting others by enhancing empathy, patience, consistency, use of listening, valuing of unstructured time in interactions, and following a service user-driven approach. In addition to self-disclosure regarding mental health, peer providers explicitly disclose other life experiences, such as those pertaining to culture, physical health, housing instability, and other life challenges (e.g., parental loss, separation from children), when supporting others. One peer provider describes the range of hardships that individuals with mental illness experience and emphasizes how sharing of experiences is multidimensional and tailored to the individual:

> [we share] to let them know that we relate and how we overcame our obstacles...That we have something in common...I don't go and just start off telling war stories...I do it more one-on-one, if a person is sharing about a traumatic experience that they've been through...what I'll do, it depends on the situation...somebody, that they've been sexually abused...I can share how I relate...People with drug and alcohol issues...Or especially working with women, relationships, and stuff like that. So it varies from person to person.

Finally, shared experience does not presume that individuals will indeed have the *same* experience. As one person receiving peer-delivered services explained, "Even if we didn't have things in common and she shared her personal history, it would make me feel more comfortable...We may not have gone through the same thing, but at least I would know that she had some struggles too, even if they weren't the same."

Research on Peer Support in Mental Health

Generally, studies find that peer support is associated with positive outcomes, performing as well as more clinical or other types of services along many outcomes, and often having an advantage in improving factors associated with recovery processes (e.g., hope, empowerment, self-efficacy) [1, 8]. Benefits of mutual support include the opportunity to learn from role models, develop new coping skills, and exchange information about available services and resources [48]. Beyond instrumental and informational support, participants report greater hope and control over their lives and reduced stigma and social isolation [48]. Participation in mutual support groups is also associated with improved psychological and social functioning (e.g., reductions in depressive symptoms and improved management of mental health) [33]. In terms of factors associated with participation in mutual support, one study of self-help groups for serious mental illness found that affiliation, acquisition of coping skills, and improved mental health were common motivators of participation, while having scheduling conflicts and feeling the groups were too "negative" (i.e., content was depressing or feeling that peers were complaining) or not helpful were common reasons for stopping [26].

Though peer-run organizations are far less studied than other forms of peer support, preliminary research suggests that participation in these organizations (either in conjunction with traditional mental health services or as a stand-alone service) is associated with positive outcomes for members/participants [15]. For example, one randomized clinical trial found that individuals experiencing an acute psychiatric crisis who were randomized to a peer-run program had fewer psychiatric symptoms and greater treatment satisfaction than their counterparts randomized to a psychiatric inpatient unit [20]. In addition to finding that peer-run organizations have more equitable structures and offer increased support and opportunities for autonomy, self-determination, social participation, and decision-making relative to mainstream organizations, they have also demonstrated greater reductions in self-stigma [37].

Peer-delivered services have been studied most extensively, with several studies finding that these peer support services are associated with lower emergency mental health service utilization rates (e.g., decreased hospitalizations and length of inpatient stay) and increased engagement in care, behavioral activation, empowerment, belonging, hopefulness, and satisfaction with, and/or quality of, different aspects of life [7, 8, 12, 16]. Further, many studies report that participants view their peer specialists as role models, increasing their hopefulness and motivation to engage in recovery, and develop better illness management skills, oftentimes as a result of peers' disclosure of their own experiences managing illness [45]. Additionally, participants express feeling more at ease with and connected to peer specialists than non-peer staff due to their shared experience of mental illness and recovery [45].

While much of the research on peer support in mental health offers support for positive outcomes, the evidence base is constrained by a lack of rigorous research, including lower-quality study designs, lack of specificity in describing peer supports and contexts being studied, high risk of bias, lack of theoretical models, and wide variability in outcome measurement making comparisons across studies difficult [25]. This has led to some inconsistent findings and calls for strengthening the evidence for peer support in mental health [25].

Development of Peer Workforce and Funding

Peer Certification and Training

To date, there is no national credentialing organization for peer certification, leaving it to the discretion of individual states – 48 of whom offer peer certification – to establish local training and standards, which vary significantly [23, 27, 31]. While there is no national standard, the Substance Abuse and Mental Health Services Administration (SAMHSA) [43]. developed a list of competencies as integral to peer support: the ability to develop collaborative, working relationships; provide support; self-disclosure of shared experience; individualization of services; assist in recovery planning; and provide linkages to community resources, advocacy, and self-development. In peer support training, many peer providers have also been trained to facilitate standardized interventions. For these interventions, it is important that training and supervision does not overemphasize technical proficiency and outcomes to be achieved, at the expense of peer specialists' unique approach and focus [44]. Such training and supervision needs to place equal emphasis on collaborating with peer specialists to promote an experiential approach, lay language, and attention to processes of care (e.g., quality of rapport, support of service user autonomy) [44].

Workforce/Workplace Integration

With the increase in peer providers, studies have examined how peer providers are integrated within organizations and the workforce [6, 17, 24]. Understanding how to facilitate such integration is particularly important given that peers often report challenging workplace contexts in mainstream settings:

> there are people from counselors on up to the clinicians who are not willing to accept us. Either they think we're tryin' to step on their toes, they think we're tryin' to take their jobs, or they think we're tryin' to be them…the problem is working with the other members of the teams outside [the peer program] and getting them to acknowledge us and to embrace us.

Challenges often include lack of clarity from both peer and non-peer staff regarding the peer role, value, and function; inadequate support and supervision; lower pay; and limited opportunities for professional development and career advancement [11, 13, 16]. Strategies for improving role clarity, as well as facilitating buy-in among non-peer staff, include formalizing roles and responsibilities, ongoing deliberations regarding roles and rationales behind responsibilities, and agency-wide trainings on the function and value of peer support work. Facilitating peers' access to peer colleagues and peer networks both within and outside an organization (e.g., peer support community of practice) is also necessary.

Formal and informal supervision should reinforce the value of the peer specialist's role and uses a collaborative approach that actively fosters and incorporates peer input [44]. Support from at least one supervisor who also identifies as a peer is beneficial [38]. Organizations should also assist peer providers with training in workplace skills (e.g., maintaining a work calendar) [44], professional development (e.g., presenting at conferences, attending trainings, leadership roles), and fostering inclusion of peer voice beyond frontline services [45]. One peer describes a positive workforce integration outcome:

> being part of a team: doctors, clinicians, PhDs, and I'm equal. I have a say. And I'm outspoken quite a bit...It's just knowing that real life experience with their school experience becomes a different way we can approach clients and that's nice.

Indeed, studies have demonstrated that working as a provider benefits peers themselves, including increased confidence, self-efficacy, self-esteem, personal growth, and community integration [9, 14, 30, 41]; lower service utilization (e.g., reduced hospitalization, emergency department visits); and reduced reliance on government entitlements [36].

Funding

Since peer-delivered mental health services first became reimbursable through Medicaid in Georgia in 1999, the Centers for Medicare and Medicaid Services have expanded funding to 41 states [31]. With the implementation of the Affordable Care Act (ACA) and its emphasis on integrated models of person-centered care, new funding opportunities have been made available for peer services in integrated primary and behavioral care settings for all states [31]. However, funding often remains a significant barrier, particularly for peer-run organizations, who struggle to preserve their autonomy while securing sustainable funding. For example, Medicaid/managed care reimbursement may require introducing stringent requirements for services that conflict with core principles [32]. Unlike other forms of peer support, mutual support groups often require little, if any, financial support from outside organizations and are generally self-sustained by members [3].

Conclusion and Future Directions

Peer support for mental health exists for a wide range of needs and is offered in a variety of formats, settings, and modalities. It has been associated with a range of positive outcomes, including reduced stigma and increased hope, sense of connectedness, empowerment, and recovery. To further broaden peer support, expansion and evaluation of peer support in more settings, as well as through virtual and social media platforms, will be essential to meeting the needs of a wider range of individuals. As peer-delivered services expand, calls for developing uniform practice standards will increase [31]. A main challenge will be ensuring that these standards promote and sustain the unique, flexible, and individualized aspects of peer supports. Expanding the types of organizations in which peer support is available will also require implementing practices that promote the work, value, and integration of peers.

Future research should incorporate more rigorous study designs and include richer descriptions of peer roles, supports offered, and the types of settings in which the support is occurring, for example, for mutual support, the degree of mutuality and reciprocity among members and type of support exchanged; for peer-run organizations, the degree to which they use a nonhierarchical approach and bilateral decision-making; and for peer-delivered services, the degree to which peer providers are offering support that differs in content and approach from non-peer providers. Especially for peer roles in mainstream mental health settings, there is a continuing need to evaluate implementation strategies, supports, and resources that will facilitate the integration of peers. Studies should also promote greater inclusion of peers on research teams and as members of advisory committees or stakeholder groups providing formal input into research activities. Significant gaps include documenting the impact of peer-run organizations and specifying the unique contributions of peer support and the mechanisms underlying their connection to positive outcomes. Finally, it is necessary to advocate for the expansion of funding and reimbursement mechanisms for peer-run organizations and peer-delivered services that can further promote their implementation and sustainability without sacrificing flexibility, autonomy, and individualized supports. Organizational and systems-level advocacy is also needed to increase salaries for peer roles and expand opportunities for career advancement and leadership.

References

1. Bellamy C, Schmutte T, Davidson L. An update on the growing evidence base for peer support. Ment Health Soc Incl. 2017;21(3):161–7.
2. Bochicchio L, Stefancic A, Gurdak K, Swarbrick M, Cabassa LJ. "We're All in this Together": peer-specialist contributions to a healthy lifestyle intervention for people with serious mental illness. Adm Policy Ment Health Ment Health Serv Res. 2019;46(3):298–310.
3. Brown LD, Shepherd MD, Wituk SA, Meissen G. Introduction to the special issue on mental health self-help. Am J Community Psychol. 2008;42(1-2):105–9.
4. Burke E, Pyle M, Machin K, Varese F, Morrison AP. The effects of peer support on empowerment, self-efficacy, and internalized stigma: a narrative synthesis and meta-analysis. Stigma and Health. 2019;4(3):337–56.
5. Cabassa LJ, Camacho D, Vélez-Grau CM, Stefancic A. Peer-based health interventions for people with serious mental illness: a systematic literature review. J Psychiatr Res. 2017;84:80–9.
6. Cabral L, Strother H, Muhr K, Sefton L, Savageau J. Clarifying the role of the mental health peer specialist in Massachusetts, USA: insights from peer specialists, supervisors and clients. Health & Social Care in the Community. 2014;22(1):104–12.
7. Chapman S, Blash L, Chan K. The peer provider workforce in behavioral health: a landscape analysis. San Francisco: UCSF Health Workforce Research Center on Long-Term Care; 2015.
8. Chinman M, George P, Dougherty RH, Daniels AS, Ghose SS, Swift A, Delphin-Rittmon ME. Peer support services for individuals with serious mental illnesses: assessing the evidence. Psychiatr Serv. 2014;65(4):429–41.
9. Colson PW, Francis LE. Consumer staff and the role of personal experience in mental health services. Soc Work Ment Health. 2009;7:385–401.
10. Cook JA, Copeland ME, Corey L, et al. Developing the evidence base for peer-led services: changes among participants following Wellness Recovery Action Planning (WRAP) education in two statewide initiatives. Psychiatr Rehabil J. 2010;34(2):113–20.

11. Daniels AS, Ashenden P, Goodale L, Stevens T. National survey of compensation among peer support specialists. 2016. The College for Behavioral Health Leadership. https://www.leaders4health.org/images/uploads/files/PSS_Compensation_Report.pdf
12. Davidson L, Guy K. Peer support among persons with severe mental illnesses: a review of evidence and experience. World Psychiatry. 2012;11(2):123–8.
13. Davis JK. Supervision of peer specialists in community mental health centers: practices that predict role clarity. Soc Work Ment Health. 2015;13(2):145–58.
14. Doherty I, Craig T, Attafua G, Boocock A, Jamieson-Craig R. The consumer-employee as a member of a mental health assertive outreach team. II. Impressions of consumer-employees and other team members. J Ment Health. 2004;13:71–81.
15. Doughty C, Tse S. Can consumer-led mental health services be equally effective? An integrative review of CLMH services in high-income countries. Community Ment Health J. 2011;47(3):252–66.
16. Gagne CA, Finch WL, Myrick KJ, Davis LM. Peer workers in the behavioral and integrated health workforce: opportunities and future directions. Am J Prev Med. 2018;54(6):S258.
17. Gates LB, Akabas SH. Developing strategies to integrate peer providers into the staff of mental health agencies. Admin Pol Ment Health. 2007;34(3):293.
18. Gidugu V, Rogers ES, Harrington S, Maru M, Johnson G, Cohee J, Hinkel J. Individual peer support: a qualitative study of mechanisms of its effectiveness. Community Ment Health J. 2015;51(4):445–52.
19. Goldstrom ID, Campbell J, Rogers JA, Lambert DB, Blacklow B, Henderson MJ, Manderscheid RW. National estimates for mental health mutual support groups, self-help organizations, and consumer-operated services. Adm Policy Ment Health Ment Health Serv Res. 2006;33(1):92–103.
20. Greenfield TK, Stoneking BC, Humphreys K, Sundby E, Bond J. A randomized trial of a mental health consumer-managed alternative to civil commitment for acute psychiatric crisis. Am J Community Psychol. 2008;42(1-2):135–44.
21. Hayes JF, Marston L, Walters K, King MB, Osborn DP. Mortality gap for people with bipolar disorder and schizophrenia: UK-based cohort study 2000–2014. Br J Psychiatry. 2017;211(3):175–81.
22. Jacobson N, Trojanowski L, Dewa CS. What do peer support workers do? A job description. BMC Health Serv Res. 2012;12(1):205.
23. Klee A, Chinman M, Kearney L. Peer specialist services: new frontiers and new roles. Psychol Serv. 2019;16(3):353–9.
24. Kuhn W, Bellinger J, Stevens-Manser S, Kaufman L. Integration of peer specialists working in mental health service settings. Commun Ment Health J. 2015;51(4):453–8.

25. Lloyd-Evans B, Mayo-Wilson E, Harrison B, Istead H, Brown E, Pilling S, et al. A systematic review and meta-analysis of randomised controlled trials of peer support for people with severe mental illness. BMC Psychiatry. 2014;14(1):39.
26. Markowitz FE. Involvement in mental health self-help groups and recovery. Health Sociol Rev. 2015;24(2):199–212.
27. Marill MC. Beyond twelve steps, peer-supported mental health care. Health Aff. 2019;38(6):896–901.
28. McGuire AB, Kukla M, Green A, Gilbride D, Mueser KT, Salyers MP. Illness management and recovery: a review of the literature. Psychiatr Serv. 2014;65(2):171–9.
29. Mental Health America. The Peer Workforce. n.d. Available from https://www.mhanational.org/peer-workforce.
30. Miyamoto Y, Sono T. Lessons from peer support among individuals with mental health difficulties: a review of the literature. Clin Pract Epidemiol Ment Health. 2012;8:22–9.
31. Myrick K, del Vecchio P. Peer support services in the behavioral healthcare workforce: State of the field. Psychiatr Rehabil J. 2016;39(3):197–203.
32. Ostrow L, Hayes SL. Leadership and characteristics of nonprofit mental health peer-run organizations nationwide. Psychiatr Serv. 2015;66(4):421–5.
33. Pistrang N, Barker C, Humphreys K. Mutual help groups for mental health problems: a review of effectiveness studies. Am J Community Psychol. 2008;42(1-2):110–21.
34. Pratt R, MacGregor A, Reid S, Given L. Wellness Recovery Action Planning (WRAP) in self-help and mutual support groups. Psychiatr Rehabil J. 2012;35(5):403–5.
35. Repper J, Carter T. A review of the literature on peer support in mental health services. J Ment Health. 2011;20(4):392–411.
36. Salzer MS, Darr N, Calhoun G, et al. Benefits of working as a certified peer specialist: results from a statewide survey. Psychiatr Rehabil J. 2013;36(3):219.
37. Scholz B, Gordon S, Happell B. Consumers in mental health service leadership: a systematic review. Int J Ment Health Nurs. 2017;26(1):20–31.
38. Silver J, Nemec PB. The role of the peer specialists: unanswered questions. Psychiatr Rehabil J. 2016;39(*3*):*289*–91.
39. Solomon P. Peer support/peer provided services underlying processes, benefits, and critical ingredients. Psychiatr Rehabil J. 2004;27(4):392–401.
40. Stefancic A, House S, Bochicchio L, Harney-Delehanty B, Osterweil S, Cabassa L. "What We Have in Common": a qualitative analysis of shared experience in peer-delivered services. Community Ment Health J. 2019;55(6):907–15.

41. Straughan H, Buckenham M. In-sight: an evaluation of user-led, recovery-based, holistic group training for bipolar disorder. J Public Ment Health. 2006;5:29–43.
42. U.S. Department of Health and Human Services, Substance Abuse and Mental Health Services Administration. Working Definition of Recovery. 2012. Retrieved from https://store.samhsa.gov/sites/default/files/d7/priv/pep12-recdef.pdf.
43. U.S. Department of Health and Human Services, Substance Abuse and Mental Health Services Administration. Core competencies for peer workers in behavioral health services. 2015. Retrieved from http://www.samhsa.gov/sites/default/files/programs_campaigns/brss_tacs/corecompetencies.pdf.
44. Vélez-Grau C, Stefancic A, Cabassa LJ. Keeping the peer in peer specialist when implementing evidence-based interventions. Health Soc Work. 2018;44(1):57–60.
45. Walker G, Bryant W. Peer support in adult mental health services: a meta-synthesis of qualitative findings. Psychiatr Rehabil J. 2013;36(1):28–34.
46. Walker ER, McGee RE, Druss BG. Mortality in mental disorders and global disease burden implications: a systematic review and meta-analysis. JAMA Psychiatry. 2015;72(4):334–41.
47. World Health Organization. Mental Disorders. 2019. Retrieved from https://www.who.int/news-room/fact-sheets/detail/mental-disorders.
48. Worrall H, Schweizer R, Marks E, Yuan L, Lloyd C, Ramjan R. The effectiveness of support groups: a literature review. Ment Health Soc Incl. 2018;22(2):85–93.

Peer Support for Chronic Medical Conditions

Megan Evans, Timothy Daaleman, and Edwin B. Fisher

Introduction

Chronic diseases are medical conditions that last 1 year or more and require ongoing medical care, or limit activities of daily living, or both [1] and are the leading causes of death and disability worldwide [2]. Many chronic diseases are tied to behavioral and lifestyle risk factors both in their etiology and course. These include tobacco use and exposure to secondhand smoke, poor nutrition, lack of physical activity, and excessive alcohol use [1]. Due to the ongoing nature and the challenges associated with managing chronic diseases, individuals often need help that augments health care and support to manage their condition effectively. Research shows that peer support can contribute to this management. This chapter describes the key functions of peer

---

M. Evans · E. B. Fisher
Department of Health Behavior, Peers for Progress, Gillings School of Global Public Health, University of North Carolina at Chapel Hill, Chapel Hill, NC, USA
e-mail: sundeme@live.unc.edu; fishere@email.unc.edu

T. Daaleman (✉)
Department of Family Medicine, School of Medicine, University of North Carolina at Chapel Hill, Chapel Hill, NC, USA
e-mail: tim_daaleman@med.unc.edu

support, the evidence base in chronic illness, and approaches for implementing peer support in chronic illness care.

Peer support refers to the provision of emotional, informational, instrumental, and appraisal support by a non-professional who shares a lived experience with those they help [3, 4]. It relies on non-hierarchical, often reciprocal relationships. In chronic disease contexts, this may take the form of a person who has been diagnosed with and is currently effectively managing their chronic condition (e.g., diabetes) while providing support to someone who also has that condition. Shared lived experience, though, may also be based on other characteristics such as being retired, widowed, or living in the same neighborhood [4, 5]. Peer supporters can serve as role models, facilitating the sharing of experiential knowledge that professionals may not have in common with their patients and often lack the time to communicate [4]. Peer support may also be provided to caregivers of those who have a chronic condition [4]. Providers of peer support are known in different settings by many different names, including "peer supporters," "community health workers" (CHWs), "promotores de salud," and "lay health workers." In the USA, "peer support" is often associated with mental health peer support specialists and CHWs with support for physical health, even though the Affordable Care Act promotes integration of behavioral health and primary care. Peer support has been broadly applied across different patient populations, health conditions, stages of disease, and settings to achieve a variety of health outcomes [6]. Employing a range of modalities (e.g., face-to-face, group-based, telephone-based, digital health), peer support may be adapted to the unique needs of its organizational home and population focus [4, 7, 8].

Five Key Functions of Peer Support

In seeking to promote peer support worldwide, *Peers for Progress* (peersforprogress.org) with which the authors are affiliated has emphasized five key functions of peer support [9, 10], following a strategy of standardization by function, not content. This provides a structure of the key functions while allowing for the adaptation and tailoring for implementation in distinct cultures, settings, and among diverse populations [11, 12]. The key functions include:

- *Being there*
  - Providing human connection or "just being there" is identified as a fundamental feature of peer support. This personal connection facilitates the basis on which peer support services are provided and has been identified as important in and of itself. In many different languages and cultures, there is an equivalent saying to "It wasn't anything she said or did, it was just knowing she was there" [13]. This expression of unconditional support may be more visible in less hierarchical and formal relationships, such as those between peer supporters and their clients, rather than in a formal provider-patient relationship.
- *Assistance in daily management*
  - For many individuals with chronic health conditions, understanding and implementing the care plans developed by health-care providers is often daunting. Medical appointments are often brief and can involve numerous and potentially complicated treatment recommendations for the patient. Peer supporters help individuals translate what physicians and other health-care providers recommend into specific, actionable plans [14]. In other words, medical providers help patients to figure out *what to do*, while peer supporters help them to figure out *how to do it* [15]. Additionally, they can help to identify barriers to effective self-management behaviors and craft ways to address these barriers.
- *Social and emotional support to promote disease self-management and coping with negative emotions*
  - Maintaining motivation for self-management is not an easy task for patients, and there are often times when support and encouragement are needed. Peer supporters can provide an opportunity for patient to share emotions and feelings [14]. Social and emotional support may also help individuals to cope with the reality of chronic disease and the distress that

may accompany it. Peer supporters can assist people with chronic medical conditions to problem-solve and overcome social and emotional barriers to sustaining evidence-based self-management behaviors [16].

- *Linkage to clinical care and community resources*
  - Peer supporters help patients recognize when they should access their health-care providers and can facilitate the timely linkage to services [17]. Additionally, peer supporters can share knowledge of other community resources that might be beneficial to patients as they navigate dealing with not only their chronic disease but also the stresses and problems associated with daily life. These resources may include health-care services, behavioral health services, community-based programs, and resources tied to social determinants such as places to buy healthy food or safe, attractive places for physical activity.
- *Ongoing support because chronic disease is for the rest of one's life*
  - As chronic disease extends over time, peer support is ideally extended over time and not time-limited. Although using peers to teach time-limited courses [18] or to promote preventive services screenings and immunizations [19] is important, the focus of peer support is to encourage the ongoing behaviors and lifestyle activities that contribute to healthy living for the rest of an individual's life. Sustained relationships can confer benefits throughout the different stages of both disease course and life course.

A Socioecological Model of Peer Support for Chronic Medical Conditions

Figure 3.1 presents a model that emphasizes that individuals are nested within interpersonal, organizational, community, and policy environments; health behavior interventions should focus on changes at more than one level if they are to be effective [20]. Peer

3 Peer Support for Chronic Medical Conditions

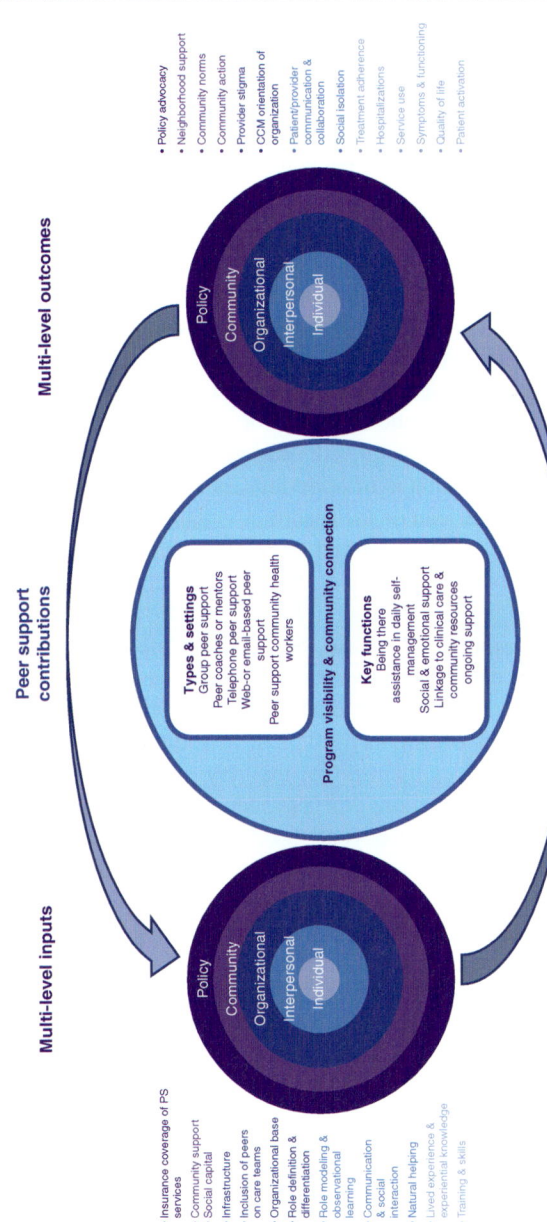

Fig. 3.1 Socioecological model of peer support for chronic medical conditions

support has inputs that span the levels of the socioecological model. Policies endorsing peer support, such as insurance coverage of CHW and peer support specialist services, allow for the provision and expansion of peer support. In addition, community and organizational capacity enable the promotion of peer support services. On the interpersonal level, peer supporters act as role models for those they serve and provide valuable social interaction. Individual peer supporters bring their unique lived experience, training, and skills to their work with patients.

These multi-level inputs contribute to the actual provision of peer support services. From the perspective of the socioecological model, peer support for chronic disease management can occur in a variety of modalities and settings. For example, it can develop organically in group medical visits and patient education classes, as patients take advantage of opportunities to share their experiences. On the other end of the spectrum, organized peer support, with volunteers or state-certified CHWs, can provide individual counseling, support daily self-management of chronic diseases, connect patients with social services, and provide a basic level of care coordination. In each case, peer support provides ongoing assistance and emotional support in chronic disease management and helps to connect individuals with appropriate care and resources in their community [21, 22]. In addition to the actual peer support services themselves, the very existence, visibility, and community connections of a peer support program can impact people and environments, beyond those directly receiving the services. By putting faces to the experience of living with a chronic medical condition and impacting norms around help-seeking and self-management behaviors, peer support can effect changes in organizations, communities, and policies.

Peer support also has multi-level impacts and outcomes. Peer support acknowledges models of individuals' vulnerabilities, but also their ability to help each other. This may promote community norms around the acknowledgement of chronic diseases and the expectations of seeking help and support for managing them. In this way, peer support can mitigate the stigmatizing belief that health problems are private issues to be dealt with only with professional health-care providers in medical settings. At the organizational level, embedding peer supporters in medical practice settings, where patients receive their care, brings an important, lived experience perspective to the care team [3]. This approach has the potential to facilitate organizational change toward a more patient-centered and collaborative care model. On the interpersonal level, peer support addresses the very real phenomenon of social isolation and provides needed support to those living with chronic medical conditions. For individuals, support from their peer mentors can help them modify their health habits, such as diet, exercise, sleep, and adherence to treatment regiments. These outcomes can also increase the capacity for peer support on multiple levels, creating a positive feedback loop where positive outcomes lead to stronger inputs and vice versa.

Evidence Base of Peer Support in Chronic Illness

There is a substantial evidence base for peer support across a wide variety of health problems, health behaviors, and support modalities. A review by Viswanathan and colleagues [23] focused on peer support provided by community health workers. It found moderate evidence of peer support's impacts on knowledge, health behaviors, utilization, and cost/cost-effectiveness. In another review, Gibbons and Tyus [24] reported efficacy in enhancing outcomes across mammography, cervical cancer screening, and a variety of other preventive services for underserved groups in US-based peer support programs. Perry and colleagues [25] identified contributions of community health workers to basic health needs in low-income countries (e.g., reducing childhood undernutrition), to primary care and health promotion in middle-income countries, and to disease management in the USA and other high-income countries.

A 2015 review conducted by the UK-based Nesta Health Lab and National Voices examined over 1000 studies of peer support provided by a wide range of individuals for a variety of health conditions to diverse population groups. It found benefits for those with long-term physical health conditions in the area of experience and emotions, behavior and health outcomes, and health costs and service use [26]. Additionally, a qualitative meta-synthesis of peer support interventions in chronic disease care reported that peer mentors' instruction had a higher impact than the provision of information alone because of its grounding in personal experience and shared identity [27].

A comprehensive review conducted through Peers for Progress [28] included peer support interventions from around the globe, addressing a wide variety of prevention and health objectives entailing sustained behavior change, as is often needed in chronic disease self-management. The review included 65 papers from the USA (34 papers) and Canada [7]; 4 from each of Bangladesh, England, Pakistan, and Scotland; and 1 from each of Australia, Brazil, Denmark, Ireland, Mozambique, New Zealand, South Africa, and Uganda. Fifty-three were from World Bank designated high-income countries and 12 from low-income, low-middle, and high-middle-income countries. The 65 papers addressed a variety of health conditions including drug, alcohol, and tobacco use disorders (3 papers), cardiovascular disease [10], diabetes [9], HIV/AIDS [6], other chronic diseases [12], maternal and child health [17], and mental health [8]. The papers also addressed both prevention [26] and disease management [29].

Across all 65 papers, 54 (83.1%) reported significant positive impacts of peer support, 40 (61.5%) reporting between-group differences (i.e., peer support compared with usual care) and another 14 (21.5%) reporting significant within-group changes (i.e., changes from pre-intervention to post-intervention). When limited to papers reporting randomized controlled trials or other controlled designs, and utilizing objective or standardized outcome measures, results were similar. Among the 43 studies meeting these criteria, 31 (72.1%) reported significant between-condition effects favoring peer support, and an additional 5 (11.6%) reported significant within-condition effects. Combining these, 36 of 43 (83.7%) papers reporting controlled designs using objective or standardized measures reported significant effects of peer support. Specific to chronic disease care, 9 of 10 papers (90%) showed positive impacts of peer support in cardiovascular disease, 8 of 9 in diabetes (88.9%), 5 of 6 (83.3%) in HIV/AIDS, and 9 of 12 (75%) in other chronic diseases. Among

19 reviews of peer support included in this systematic review, a median of 64.5% of studies reviewed reported significant positive effects of peer support.

Engaging the Hardly Reached

Those who experience disproportionate, avoidable, and high-cost care are often not reached by clinical and preventive services. Peer support may be most successful among these "hardly reached" groups with whom one might expect least success, due to individual (e.g., psychological distress), demographic (e.g., ethnic minority), or cultural-environmental (e.g., rural) characteristics [30]. A systematic review of 47 studies of peer support for such groups often challenged to engage in health care found that 94% reported significant changes favoring peer support [30]. For example, asthma coaches were able to engage nearly 90% of mothers in a population of Medicaid-covered children who were hospitalized for asthma. The coaches sustained that engagement, averaging 21 contacts per parent over a 2-year intervention, and reducing re-hospitalization by 52% [31]. Among ethnic minority patients of safety net clinics in San Francisco [32], the impact of peer support over usual care alone was greatest among those initially identified as having low medication adherence and self-management [33]. In veterans with diabetes participating in peer support dyads [34], improvements in blood glucose were greatest among those with initially low levels of diabetes support or health literacy [35]. In Pakistan, peer support for post-partum depression was most effective relative to controls among women with household debt and/or relatively low levels of economic empowerment [36].

Reaching Populations

Most studies of peer support are based on selected samples, shedding little light on the challenge of reaching entire populations. A collaboration of Alivio Medical Center, a federally qualified health center in Chicago, UnidosUS, and Peers for Progress sought to reach the population of an estimated 3500–4000 Latino adults with type 2 diabetes served by Alivio [37]. The program, *Compañeros en Salud*, reached 88% of 471 patients categorized as high need (i.e., elevated HbA1c values and/or distress or depression and/or judged by their primary care providers as especially likely to benefit). Patients initially received biweekly phone calls, reduced to monthly, and then quarterly as progress warranted. *Compañeros* also engaged 82% of 3316 assigned to regular care that included group classes and activities and quarterly contacts via phone or during regular clinical appointments. Across all 3787 Alivio patients with diabetes, HbA1c declined from 8.22% to 8.14% over 2 years. Among high-need patients, HbA1c declined from 9.43 to 9.16%, and the proportion with moderate to good HbA1c control ($\leq 8\%$) increased from 19% to 26%.

Peer Support and the Chronic Care Model

The Chronic Care Model (CCM) has become a major framework for the delivery of chronic care services and includes several components: (1) the organization of health care, (2) delivery system design, (3) decision support, (4) clinical information systems, (5) self-management support, and (6) community resources [38, 39]. The CCM advocates for care that adheres to evidence-based guidelines and medical practices that are designed to meet the needs of patients with chronic health conditions [40, 41]. Additionally, the CCM emphasizes patient self-management and support for behavioral change, acknowledging the crucial role of the patient outside of the clinical setting [40, 41].

The effective role of peer support can be applied for each of the CCM components. The CCM is responsive to individuals' needs for social and emotional support in the management of chronic conditions, a key function of peer support. Peer support has the capacity to link clinical care and community resources, an integral feature of the CCM. In addition to helping individuals identify and gain access to care, peer support also facilitates the relationships between individuals and their care providers.

Through frequent interaction with patients and by understanding their needs, peer support can enrich the perspectives of other members of the clinical team, particularly in decision-making. Peer support can deliver culturally competent education and facilitate the adoption of self-management skills to enhance treatment adherence. Whether as part of the clinical team or as a closely linked resource, developing peer support services should include representatives of communities who receive care from those service areas. Incorporating peer support can sharpen the focus of the respective delivery system to one that is dedicated to patients' perspectives and concerns.

Examples of Peer Support and the Chronic Care Model

There are many examples of how peer support can be integrated into health-care delivery through the CCM. For example, the *Diabetes Equity Project*, a program of the Baylor Health Care System, used the CCM to integrate CHWs into primary care teams in order to address inequities in five community clinics serving low-income Latino adults with diabetes [42, 43]. As part of system redesign, CHWs were recruited from medical assistants, trained in general peer support skills and diabetes-specific information, and embedded within clinical teams. Development of the CHW role included taking on tasks from primary care providers, including diabetes education, nutrition counseling, and patient follow-up, as well as adding new tasks, such as social support and linkage to community resources. System redesign included locating CHWs in the practice setting, facilitating regular and routine interactions, including as-needed on-the-spot consultations in contrast to referrals with potential delays and uncertain completion. CHWs provided useful information to PCPs regarding their patients' needs, and patients reported that the intervention had improved their relationships with those providers [42].

A multifaceted intervention to test the CCM model for patients with macular degeneration focused on reorganization of care around trained Chronic Care Coaches (CCCs) [44, 45]. In participating clinical sites, the CCC was a practice assistant [45] trained to monitor the treatment, including telephone reminders, patient information, and direct self-management support. The CCCs assisted patients in self-management, including by monitoring patients' weekly self-administration of the Amsler test for monitoring vision and helping to develop an action plan that helped patients manage symptoms, estimate their severity, and devise response strategies in the case of deterioration. In addition, the program included planning and arranging contact between patients and physicians and a monthly structured follow-up call with the patients [44, 45].

In an intervention to reduce coronary heart disease risk among African Americans with hypertension, patients with well-controlled hypertension provided peer-based self-management support for reducing blood pressure and cardiovascular risk through three bimonthly telephone calls from peer supporters with well-controlled hypertension as well as practice-based office support on alternate months. The content of calls included healthy diet, exercise, medication adherence, and smoking cessation. To coordinate care, peer supporters left voicemail messages to clinical staff reporting concerns to be addressed in patients' clinical visits [46].

Another smoking cessation intervention employed nurses to provide initial education and counseling to hospitalized patients who, after discharge, received follow-up telephone counseling from a quit-line counselor [47]. For those patients who were ambivalent about quitting, the counselor focused on increasing motivation to quit. For those patients who remained committed to quitting, the counselor focused on relapse prevention. The quit-line counselors encouraged follow-up with primary care providers upon discharge.

A comprehensive program in a federally qualified health center improved glycemic control among a population of mostly Latino adults with diabetes [48]. Assistance in daily management took place through a variety of activities that included a weekly breakfast club that highlighted nutrition and cooking skills using healthy modifications of traditional Puerto Rican recipes; a weekly drop-in afternoon snack club in which patients were taught how to prepare healthy snacks and interact with other patients and staff to reinforce problem-solving and self-management skills; diabetes education classes; chronic disease self-management classes [49] facilitated by CHWs; daily, on-site exercise classes; and bilingual/bicultural CHW services provided directly to patients.

Approaches to Implementing Peer Support

Peer Support in Health-Care Settings

Peer support can be integrated into health-care systems, extending the reach of hospitals and other health-care systems beyond the clinical care provided within them [50]. One approach to reaching populations with peer support is the integration of peer support into primary care and patient-centered medical homes [50]. Clinicians or other health-care team members can identify patients who are skilled at and have demonstrated success in the self-management of their medical conditions to potentially serve as peer supporters. Peer supporters may be integrated into the care team or serve to extend the role of the clinical case manager.

Employing peer supporters as an integral part of a care team facilitates important communication and linkage between patients and their medical providers. The earlier described program involving macular degeneration using Chronic Care Coaches included planning and arranging contact between patients and physicians and a monthly structured follow-up call with the patients [44, 45]. As noted in the model from the Baylor Health Care System, CHWs provided useful information to PCPs regarding their patients' needs; patients reported that the intervention had improved their relationships with those providers [42]. Similarly, in the intervention for African American patients with hypertension [46], peer supporters left voicemail messages to clinical staff reporting concerns to be addressed in patients' clinical visits.

Integrating Behavioral Health and Peer Support

Chronic diseases are often accompanied by psychosocial and mental health problems, including depression and anxiety disorders [51]. A broad range of factors influence psychological and physical health, from epigenetic effects of adverse or positive aspects of early development to social and economic contexts of family and social relationships and organizational, economic, and cultural factors. Those disadvantaged across these developmental, biological, and psychosocial determinants [51] are likely to experience both physical and psychological problems and disproportionate emergency and hospital care. The importance of social contact and emotional support [52] suggests that simple, frequent, and affirming peer support may be especially helpful to those with emotional distress.

In a Hong Kong study, peer support reduced distress and related hospitalizations among adults with diabetes. Among the 20% of patients who reported heightened depression, anxiety, and/or stress, peer support both improved distress scores and reduced hospitalizations (relative risk = 0.15) relative to controls, reducing overall hospitalizations to the level of those low on distress measures [53]. That the peer support was designed to focus on diabetes management, not to reduce emotional distress, suggests the implicit value of "being there" as in the first of the five key functions discussed earlier.

Peer Support and Health Information Technologies

Several health information modalities (e.g., computer, mobile, and web-based technology) have been studied for their potential to enhance, extend, and scale up peer support. These platforms create environments for the exchange of unstructured and/or structured peer support, provide patient education, encourage self-management behaviors, and collect and analyze patient health data to deliver personalized messages and guide clinical decision-making. Health information technologies (HIT) are able to respond in real-time, delivering support that is contextual, accessible, and convenient. Some people prefer these modalities because they allow for the exchange of rich, thoughtful information and are unique avenues of self-expression. Additionally, HIT can facilitate peer support across geographic distances, enabling those with rare diseases to find others with the same condition, improving access to support and affordability of care.

In remote areas of Australia, for example, Telephone Linked Care [54] provided messages and reminders that were personalized according to individual self-management and clinical measures, all monitored through data entered through patients' smartphones. HbA1c values declined from 8.8% to 8.0% and were accompanied by improvements on quality-of-life indicators that exceeded those in a control condition. Medication costs were lower as well ($1542 versus $1821 on average). Users reported substantial social and emotional support; 79% strongly agreed that it gave them confidence to manage their diabetes better [55].

Online communities (e.g., forums, social media) are frequently consumer-driven networks whose purpose is to facilitate the exchange of peer support while providing linkages to health-care professionals [56]. These online communities can be responsive to the needs of their members, leading to high levels of satisfaction. One review concluded that computer-mediated environments enhance an individual's ability to interact with peers while increasing the convenience of obtaining personalized support [57]. Aspects of mobile phone interventions (e.g., text messaging, mobile apps, biometrics) can offer interactive features, monitoring tools, and personalized feedback to enhance the quality of peer support interactions [58].

A pilot test of a lay health coaching intervention was enhanced with a diabetes self-management application (BlueStar™) [59]. The intervention involved health coaches who provided telephone-based diabetes self-management support and encouraged the routine use of BlueStar for day-to-day self-management tasks. Patient-generated data in BlueStar was shared with the health coaches and a nurse care coordinator to guide highly personalized care. Both intervention components proactively engaged with participants to achieve high rates of retention and overall program satisfaction. Patients who participated in this intervention made behavior changes and experienced a significant drop in HbA1c. One finding from this project was the significant correlation between total entries in BlueStar and total coach contacts, which suggests complementary roles between health coaching and the diabetes application.

High tech can complement and facilitate, but does not replace, the soft touch of peer support. Offering both peer support and digital health can promote patient choice, depending on the support they need or prefer. Digital health technologies can address the routine tasks and monitoring needed for chronic disease self-management, leaving peer supporters to provide highly individualized support for more complex problems. These platforms can extend peer support to more people and integrate the efficiencies of high tech with the humanizing force of personal contact [60]. Investigators are particularly interested in integrating digital health technologies for peer supporters that have the capacity to generate actionable data; prompt timely, context-sensitive outreach; and guide decision-making [61]. Such programs may have the capacity to reach entire populations while maximizing the efforts of peer supporters and clinical staff.

Conclusion

Peer support for chronic disease management can be implemented in many different forms and settings. Underlying the numerous examples of successful peer support programs outlined in this chapter are the five key functions of peer support: being there, assistance in daily self-management, social and emotional support, linkage to clinical and community resources, and ongoing support. This standardization by function, not content, allows for peer support programs to be designed and implemented in ways that accommodate a diverse array of organizational, community, and cultural settings. Tailoring peer support programs to target the key factors identified as critically important to different health conditions, care settings, and patient populations make peer support programs adaptive to the needs of those they serve. Reflecting the socioecological perspective introduced here, peer support programs may have an effect at the level of organizations and systems, supporting the transition in medicine from a focus on medical treatment to integrating the lived experience of patients and promoting chronic disease self-management. Implementation approaches include integration with hospitals, primary care settings, behavioral health, and use of technology to promote better self-management among people with chronic health problems.

References

1. Centers for Disease Control and Prevention. About Chronic Diseases 2019 [updated July 30]. Available from: https://www.cdc.gov/chronicdisease/about/index.htm.
2. World Health Organization. Chronic diseases and health promotion 2019. Available from: https://www.who.int/chp/about/integrated_cd/en/.
3. Solomon P. Peer support/peer provided services underlying processes, benefits, and critical ingredients. Psychiatr Rehabil J. 2004;27(4):392.
4. Dennis C-L. Peer support within a health care context: a concept analysis. Int J Nurs Stud. 2003;40(3):321–32.
5. Fisher EB, Coufal MM, Parada H, Robinette JB, Tang PY, Urlaub DM, et al. Peer support in health care and prevention: cultural, organizational, and dissemination issues. Annu Rev Public Health. 2014;35:363–83.
6. Fisher EB, Boothroyd RI, Elstad EA, Hays L, Henes A, Maslow GR, et al. Peer support of complex health behaviors in prevention and disease management with special reference to diabetes: systematic reviews. Clin Diabetes Endocrinol. 2017;3(1):4.
7. Heisler M. Different models to mobilize peer support to improve diabetes self-management and clinical outcomes: evidence, logistics, evaluation considerations and needs for future research. Fam Pract. 2009;27(suppl_1):i23–32.
8. Heisler M. Overview of peer support models to improve diabetes self-management and clinical outcomes. Diabetes Spect. 2007;20(4):214–21.
9. Fisher EB, Boothroyd RI, Coufal MM, Baumann LC, Mbanya JC, Rotheram-Borus MJ, et al. Peer support for self-management of diabetes improved outcomes in international settings. Health Aff (Millwood). 2012;31(1):130–9.
10. Fisher EB, Earp JA, Maman S, Zolotor A. Cross-cultural and international adaptation of peer support for diabetes management. Fam Pract. 2010;27(Suppl 1):i6–i16.
11. Hawe P, Shiell A, Riley T. Complex interventions: how "out of control" can a randomised controlled trial be? BMJ. 2004;328(7455):1561–3.

12. Aro A, Smith J, Dekker J. Contextual evidence in clinical medicine and health promotion. Eur J Public Health. 2008;18(6):548.
13. Fisher EB, Bhushan NL, Coufal MM, Kowitt SD, Parada H, Sokol RL, et al. Peer support in prevention, chronic disease management, and well-being. In: Principles and concepts of behavioral medicine. New York, NY: Springer; 2018. p. 643–77.
14. Fisher EB, Boothroyd RI, Coufal MM, Baumann LC, Mbanya JC, Rotheram-Borus MJ, et al. Peer support for self-management of diabetes improved outcomes in international settings. Health Aff. 2012;31(1):130–9.
15. Davis KL, O'Toole ML, Brownson CA, Llanos P, Fisher EB. Teaching how, not what. Diabetes Educ. 2007;33(S6):208S–15S.
16. Thorpe CT, Fahey LE, Johnson H, Deshpande M, Thorpe JM, Fisher EB. Facilitating healthy coping in patients with diabetes: a systematic review. Diabetes Educ. 2013;39(1):33–52.
17. Peers for Progress, editor Global evidence for peer support: humanizing health care. Report from an International Conference hosted by Peers for Progress and the National Council of La Raza. American Academy of Family Physicians Foundation; 2014; Leawood, KS.
18. Lorig K, Ritter PL, Plant K. A disease-specific self-help program compared with a generalized chronic disease self-help program for arthritis patients. Arthritis Rheum. 2005;53(6):950–7.
19. Earp JA, Eng E, O'Malley MS, Altpeter M, Rauscher G, Mayne L, et al. Increasing use of mammography among older, rural African American women: results from a community trial. Am J Public Health. 2002;92(4):646–54.
20. Sallis JF, Owen N. Ecological models. Health Behav Health Educ Theory Res Pract. 1997;2:403–24.
21. Rosenthal EL, Brownstein JN, Rush CH, Hirsch GR, Willaert AM, Scott JR, et al. Community health workers: part of the solution. Health Aff (Millwood). 2010;29(7):1338–42.
22. Fisher EB, Coufal MM, Parada H, Robinette JB, Tang P, Urlaub D, et al. Peer support in health care and prevention: cultural, organizational and dissemination issues. In: Fielding J, Brownson RC, Green L, editors. Annu rev public health. 35. Palo Alto: Annual Reviews; 2014. p. 363–83.
23. Viswanathan M, Kraschnewski JL, Nishikawa B, Morgan LC, Honeycutt AA, Thieda P, et al. Outcomes and costs of community health worker interventions: a systematic review. Med Care. 2010;48(9):792–808.
24. Gibbons MC, Tyus NC. Systematic review of U.S.-based randomized controlled trials using community health workers. Prog Community Health Partnersh. 2007;1(4):371–81.
25. Perry HB, Zulliger R, Rogers MM. Community health workers in low-, middle-, and high-income countries: an overview of their history, recent evolution, and current effectiveness. Annu Rev Public Health. 2014;35:399–421.

26. Nesta Health Lab & National Voices. Peer support: what is it and does it work. London: Nesta and National Voices; 2015.
27. Embuldeniya G, Veinot P, Bell E, Bell M, Nyhof-Young J, Sale JE, et al. The experience and impact of chronic disease peer support interventions: a qualitative synthesis. Patient Educ Couns. 2013;92(1):3–12.
28. Fisher EB, Boothroyd RI, Elstad EA, Hays L, Henes A, Maslow GR, et al. Peer support of complex health behaviors in prevention and disease management with special reference to diabetes: systematic reviews. Clin Diabetes Endocrinol. 2017;3(4):1–23. https://doi.org/10.1186/s40842-017-0042-3.
29. Glasgow RE, Funnell MM, Bonomi AE, Davis C, Beckham V, Wagner EH. Self-management aspects of the improving chronic illness care breakthrough series: implementation with diabetes and heart failure teams. Ann Behav Med. 2002;24:80–7.
30. Sokol R, Fisher E. Peer support for the hardly reached: a systematic review. Am J Public Health. 2016;106(7):e1–8.
31. Fisher EB, Strunk RC, Highstein GR, Kelley-Sykes R, Tarr KL, Trinkaus K, et al. A randomized controlled evaluation of the effect of community health workers on hospitalization for asthma: the asthma coach. Arch Pediatr Adolesc Med. 2009;163(3):225–32.
32. Thom DH, Ghorob A, Hessler D, De Vore D, Chen E, Bodenheimer TA. Impact of peer health coaching on glycemic control in low-income patients with diabetes: a randomized controlled trial. Ann Fam Med. 2013;11(2):137–44.
33. Moskowitz D, Thom DH, Hessler D, Ghorob A, Bodenheimer T. Peer coaching to improve diabetes self-management: which patients benefit most? J Gen Intern Med. 2013;28(7):938–42.
34. Heisler M, Vijan S, Makki F, Piette JD. Diabetes control with reciprocal peer support versus nurse care management: a randomized trial. Ann Intern Med. 2010;153(8):507–15.
35. Piette JD, Resnicow K, Choi H, Heisler M. A diabetes peer support intervention that improved glycemic control: mediators and moderators of intervention effectiveness. Chronic Illn. 2013;9(4):258–67.
36. Rahman A, Sikander S, Malik A, Ahmed I, Tomenson B, Creed F. Effective treatment of perinatal depression for women in debt and lacking financial empowerment in a low-income country. Br J Psychiatry. 2012;201(6):451–7.
37. Fisher EB, Ballesteros J, Bhushan N, Coufal MM, Kowitt SD, McDonough AM, et al. Key features of peer support in chronic disease prevention and management. Health Aff (Millwood). 2015;34(9):1523–30.
38. Wagner EH, Austin BT, Davis C, Hindmarsh M, Schaefer J, Bonomi A. Improving chronic illness care: translating evidence into action. Health Aff (Millwood). 2001;20:54–78.

39. Wagner EH, Austin BT, Von Korff M. Organizing care for patients with chronic illness. Milbank Q. 1996;74:511–44.
40. Wagner EH, Austin BT, Von Korff M. Organizing care for patients with chronic illness. Milbank Q. 1996;74(4):511–44.
41. Wagner EH, Austin BT, Davis C, Hindmarsh M, Schaefer J, Bonomi A. Improving chronic illness care: translating evidence into action. Health Aff. 2001;20(6):64–78.
42. Collinsworth AW, Vulimiri M, Snead C, Walton J. Community health workers in primary care practice: redesigning health care delivery systems to extend and improve diabetes care in underserved populations. Health Promot Pract. 2014;15(2 Suppl):51S–61S.
43. Collinsworth AW, Vulimiri M, Schmidt KL, Snead CA. Effectiveness of a community health worker-led diabetes self-management education program and implications for CHW involvement in care coordination strategies. Diabetes Educ. 2013;39(6):792–9.
44. Frei A, Woitzek K, Wang M, Held U, Rosemann T. The chronic care for age-related macular degeneration study (CHARMED): study protocol for a randomized controlled trial. Trials. 2011;12:221.
45. Markun S, Dishy A, Neuner-Jehle S, Rosemann T, Frei A. The chronic care for wet age related macular degeneration (CHARMED) study: a randomized controlled trial. PLoS One. 2015;10(11):e0143085.
46. Turner BJ, Hollenbeak CS, Liang Y, Pandit K, Joseph S, Weiner MG. A randomized trial of peer coach and office staff support to reduce coronary heart disease risk in African-Americans with uncontrolled hypertension. J Gen Intern Med. 2012;27(10):1258–64.
47. Katz D, Vander Weg M, Fu S, Prochazka A, Grant K, Buchanan L, et al. A before-after implementation trial of smoking cessation guidelines in hospitalized veterans. Implement Sci. 2009;4:58.
48. Liebman J, Heffernan D, Sarvela P. Establishing diabetes self-management in a community health center serving low-income Latinos. Diabetes Educ. 2007;33(Suppl 6):132S–8S.
49. Lorig KR, Ritter PL, Gonzalez VM. Hispanic chronic disease self-management: a randomized community-based outcome trial. Nurs Res. 2003;52:361–9.
50. Daaleman TP, Fisher EB. Enriching patient-centered medical homes through peer support. Ann Fam Med. 2015;13(Suppl 1):S73–S8.
51. Fisher EB, Chan JCN, Kowitt S, Nan H, Sartorius N, Oldenburg B. Conceptual perspectives on the co-occurrence of mental and physical disease: diabetes and depression as a model. In: Sartorius N, Maj M, Holt R, editors. Comorbidity of mental and physical disorders. Basel: Karger; 2015.
52. Harlow HF, Harlow M. Learning to love. Am Sci. 1966;54:244–72.
53. Chan JC, Sui Y, Oldenburg B, Zhang Y, Chung HH, Goggins W, et al. Effects of telephone-based peer support in patients with type 2 diabetes

mellitus receiving integrated care: a randomized clinical trial. JAMA Intern Med. 2014;174(6):972–81.
54. Williams ED, Bird D, Forbes AW, Russell A, Ash S, Friedman R, et al. Randomised controlled trial of an automated, interactive telephone intervention (TLC diabetes) to improve type 2 diabetes management: baseline findings and six-month outcomes. BMC Public Health. 2012;12:602.
55. Oldenburg B. Impacts on social support and emotional wellbeing of automated "peer support". Berlin: International Society for Affective Disorders; 2014.
56. Cotter AP, Durant N, Agne AA, Cherrington AL. Internet interventions to support lifestyle modification for diabetes management: a systematic review of the evidence. J Diabetes Complicat. 2014;28(2):243–51.
57. Lewinski AA, Fisher EB. Social interaction in type 2 diabetes computer-mediated environments: how inherent features of the channels influence peer-to-peer interaction. Chronic Illn. 2016;12(2):116–44.
58. Quinn CC, Shardell MD, Terrin ML, Barr EA, Ballew SH, Gruber-Baldini AL. Cluster-randomized trial of a mobile phone personalized behavioral intervention for blood glucose control. Diabetes Care. 2011;34(9):1934–42.
59. Kowitt SD, Tang PY, Peeples M, Duni J, Peskin S, Fisher EB. Combining the high tech with the soft touch: population health management using ehealth and peer support. Popul Health Manag. 2017;20(1):3–9.
60. Lauckner HM, Hutchinson SL. Peer support for people with chronic conditions in rural areas: a scoping review. Rural Remote Health. 2016;16(1):3601.
61. Aikens JE, Zivin K, Trivedi R, Piette JD. Diabetes self-management support using mHealth and enhanced informal caregiving. J Diabetes Complicat. 2014;28(2):171–6.

Peer Support for the Bereaved

Paul T. Bartone and Chantel M. Dooley

Grief is a normal human response to death and loss. However, for some people the experience of grief can be severe and debilitating. This happens when grief goes on for too long a time or interferes with normal life functioning. Complicated grief was recognized in the early 1990s as a prolonging of the normal grief process that impairs the mental and physical health of its sufferers. While there currently is not full agreement as to its diagnostic features, it was included in DSM-5 [1] as "persistent complex bereavement disorder." Prevalence estimates for complicated grief in the general population range from a low of 2.4% to 4.8% [2–4]. Among the bereaved only population, prevalence ranges from 10% to 40% [4–8].

It's known that people who experience the death of a spouse or child are at higher risk for complicated grief, and women gener-

---

This chapter is based in part on previous reports by Bartone et al. (2018), Bartone et al. (2019), and Dooley et al. (2019).

P. T. Bartone (✉)
Institute for National Strategic Studies, National Defense University, Washington, DC, USA

C. M. Dooley
Tragedy Assistance Program for Survivors, Arlington, VA, USA
e-mail: chantel@taps.org

ally are at higher risk [2, 3]. In 2017 (the last year for which data are available), the US population at large suffered 243,039 sudden, injury-related deaths [9]. This number includes motor vehicle accidents, suicides, homicides, drug and alcohol overdoses, and poisonings. These unexpected deaths leave behind an even larger number of grieving loved ones, 10% or more of whom will experience complicated and debilitating grief.

Some groups such as the military, or others in high-risk occupations, may experience higher rates of sudden death, especially during periods of conflict and high operational activity. For example, during the 10-year period from 2001 to 2011, a total of 15,938 active duty military personnel died, and 80% of these were from sudden and traumatic causes including combat (31.5%), accidents (34.0%), and suicide (14.5%). This group of deceased service members left behind a total of 10,020 bereaved spouses and some 12,641 grieving children [10]. And when the death is sudden and violent, survivors typically have greater difficulty dealing with the loss [11, 12]. In light of all this, it is important that healthcare providers be aware of the signs and symptoms of complicated grief, as well as intervention strategies that can promote healthy grief recovery in bereaved family members and friends. Peer support-based programs are being used with increasing success to help the bereaved. This chapter will briefly review the evidence on peer support programs for the bereaved and provide some best practice guidelines based upon existing successful programs in this area.

Some Background on Peer Support

Starting around 1990 there was a dramatic increase in the use of peer support programs in the USA and elsewhere. In 2005, the number of peer providers in mental health settings was estimated at more than 10,000 in the USA alone [13]. Peer supporters are used in other domains as well, including with police, firefighters, military veterans, and people with disabilities, addictions, and chronic illnesses such as cancer and diabetes.

Peer support can be defined as "a system of giving and receiving help founded on key principles of respect, shared responsibility, and mutual agreement of what is helpful" [14]. While peer support programs can differ in many ways, they always entail people with similar backgrounds providing emotional, social, or practical support to each other [15]. Peer support services can aim, for example, to promote hope and recovery from illness or trauma and improve life skills, psychological well-being, and social integration [16]. Regardless of the specific objectives, peer supporters draw on their shared experiences in order to provide empathic understanding, information, and advice to those they are helping.

Peer support can be understood as a special form of *social support* – the belief that there are people available who are willing and able to provide emotional as well as practical support and advice [15]. Social support may include emotional support, advice and information, practical assistance, and help in understanding events [17]. Fairly extensive research shows that social support is linked to good health and positive outcomes in general, especially when people are dealing with stressful situations [18]. Social support from peers appears to be especially helpful in these cases [17, 19]. For example, a study of Vietnam veterans found that those who received more social support from peers reported less post-traumatic stress disorder (PTSD) than soldiers who were more isolated from their peers [20]. Another study of Gulf War veterans found that perceived peer social support (horizontal cohesion) and personality hardiness served to reduce the ill effects of combat exposure [21]. The benefits of peer support are thus likely due in part to the social support that this provides. In peer support programs, this effect may be enhanced due to the rapid trust that is often established in the peer-to-peer relationship [22].

What's the scientific evidence for peer support? An early report by Solomon reviewed the evidence for peer support in mental health programs and concluded there was a "very high level of support" for the effectiveness of peer providers in influencing positive outcomes for recipients [15]. Additional studies have found that self-help therapy by paraprofessionals or peers was equally effective and in some cases superior to therapy provided by professionals in reducing mental health problems such as depression [23, 24].

Studies of peer support for individuals with more severe mental health problems (i.e., schizophrenia, major affective disorder) have also found positive evidence [25, 26]. For example, Davidson et al. (1999) reported that self-help peer groups led to reduced symptoms (e.g., feeling tense or anxious, confused thinking, suicidal thoughts) and also increased social connections and quality of life for the participants [26]. A more recent review found that peer support resulted in multiple benefits for mental health patients including better compliance with treatment programs, fewer hospitalizations, and increased autonomy and a sense of hope [27].

Peer Support for the Bereaved

One area where peer support programs are being applied with increasing frequency is to help survivors who are grieving the death of a family member or friend. For example, peer support programs have been developed to facilitate grief recovery in police and emergency responders exposed to death [19]; parents who have lost a child to suicide, drugs, or illness [28]; and survivors of military death [29].

A number of studies have shown that peer support interventions can facilitate adaptation to loss in the bereaved. For example, a study of bereaved fathers in Finland found that those who received peer support showed less severe grief symptoms and more personal growth than bereaved fathers not receiving this support [30]. Other studies have documented reduced symptoms of depression and despair in bereaved survivors of a suicide death who received peer support assistance [31, 32]. Also looking at bereaved survivors of death due to suicide, Feigelman and colleagues found that peer support was associated with more personal growth and positive grief resolution [28, 33].

A recent systematic review found further evidence for the effectiveness of peer support for the bereaved [34]. Of 32 studies reviewed, a majority found evidence that peer support was helpful to the bereaved. For example, Kaunonen et al. (1999) found lower anxiety and avoidance in both widows and widowers who received peer support [35]. In another study of bereaved parents who lost a child, Worden and Silverman (1993) reported that lack of peer support was associated with increased depression [36]. Riley et al. (2007) also found fewer complicated grief symptoms in bereaved parents who received peer support [37]. Additional research shows significant reductions in depression and despair and increased personal growth in bereaved family members who received peer support [31, 32, 38].

Survivors of death by suicide may experience grief reactions that are in some ways different and perhaps more difficult to manage than those of non-suicide death survivors. Grief for suicide survivors may be complicated by feelings of shame and stigma surrounding the death, a sense of rejection and abandonment, feelings of guilt and self-blame, and self-destructive thoughts [39]. To the extent this is true, suicide survivors may benefit more from peer support that comes from other suicide survivors like themselves, rather than survivors of non-suicide deaths [29]. Indeed, several studies indicate that bereaved survivors of a suicide death benefit especially from peer support provided by others who have also experienced a suicide in their lives [31, 32, 40]. In the next section, we provide an organizational case study of a peer support program that has proven to be effective in helping bereaved survivors of a military death.

Peer Support to the Bereaved: The Tragedy Assistance Program for Survivors (TAPS)

The Tragedy Assistance Program for Survivors was first established by Bonnie Carroll shortly after her husband died in a 1992 military plane crash along with seven other servicemen. Following the crash, Carroll searched for support to help her cope with this sudden and life-changing loss. She eventually found the best support came from the other widows whose husbands died in the same crash. It was this personal experience that convinced Carroll of the power of peer support for grieving survivors and led her in 1994 to establish the Tragedy Assistance Program for Survivors (TAPS). TAPS is a nonprofit organization with the goal of providing bereavement care and peer support resources for survivors of a military death and is funded entirely through private donations [41].

Key to the TAPS approach is the use of peer support specialists, volunteers who have experienced a military death of their own and have received special training in the management of grief [42]. A central assumption behind peer support is that due to shared life experiences and circumstances, peers are better able to establish relationships of trust and support with those they are assisting [15]. Peer support provides three main benefits over traditional mental health approaches: (1) an increased sense of hope through positive self-disclosure; (2) use of similar background and experience to facilitate positive role modeling; and (3) greater trust, understanding, and empathy between the peer supporter and the recipient [43].

The TAPS model makes use of peer support in a number of programs that aim to facilitate healthy grief recovery in survivors. Drawing primarily on Worden's (2009) theoretical framework of grief recovery [44], the TAPS model of care for the bereaved consists of three broad phases: *stabilization*, *hopeful reappraisal*, and *positive integration*. These phases will be discussed in turn, along with some examples of TAPS programs that aim to assist the bereaved in each phase of grief recovery.

Stabilization

The main goal in the stabilization phase is to provide immediate care, comfort, and practical support to survivors following a sudden death. During this phase, survivors need first of all to experience a sense of safety and stability, which is provided by TAPS peer supporters. Initial contact often occurs via a telephone call to the TAPS National Military Survivor Helpline *(800-959-8277)*.

This helpline is staffed 24 hours a day, 7 days a week by fellow military survivors. Calling this helpline puts survivors in touch with care providers specifically focused on the unique circumstances survivors face after a death in the military. After some basic information is obtained, the bereaved survivor is connected to a range of programs, services, and resources as appropriate for that individual.

In addition to the TAPS internal programs, TAPS peer supporters also connect survivors with local grief support groups and mental health professionals within their local communities who can provide survivors with resources specific to their unique needs. Following initial contact and establishing some basic level of trust, survivors are assessed for potential suicide risk and clinical treatment needs. Referrals to mental health professionals are made as appropriate or when requested by the survivor. TAPS peer supporters always have licensed mental health clinicians available to consult with on any such questions.

One of the primary TAPS program interventions consists of regular seminars or "grief camps" which are held in multiple locations across the country throughout the year. These seminars provide a venue where survivors can meet and receive information on grief, bereavement, coping skills, peer-based emotional support, and related resources. TAPS also provides extensive web-based resources including text-based chat sessions, video chat sessions, blogs, and message boards where survivors can engage with TAPS staff and other survivors, have their questions answered, and share stories of their loved ones.

Survivors are often in need of advice and support on financial and administrative issues, such as applying for insurance benefits. The TAPS *Casework Advocacy team* connects with survivors to identify areas of need to include emergency financial assistance for survivors who experience hardships such as gaps in insurance coverage, emergency basic housing and utility bills, education benefits, and funeral costs. These services also provide survivors with a sense of safety and stability, freeing them to address their grief-related emotions.

Hopeful Reappraisal

The key goal in the hopeful reappraisal phase is to assist the survivor in confronting and accepting the loss, addressing emotions, and establishing a sense of hope for the future. As humans, there is a normal tendency to avoid what feels painful. For those experiencing grief, while there may be some value in emotional detachment in the early grief period, in order to move toward recovery it is critical that survivors begin to approach and confront their grief. This phase is in alignment with Worden's period of experiencing the pain of grief [44]. TAPS programs seek to facilitate the open confrontation and acceptance of loss, while at the same time encouraging feelings of hope regarding the future. As survivors begin to adjust to their new "normal," additional TAPS programs are available to support survivors through this stage of the grief process.

The TAPS *Peer Mentor* program becomes especially important during this phase. All peer mentors are volunteers and are themselves military loss survivors and are at least 1½ years past their own loss [45]. Peer mentors receive extensive training in order to prepare them for this role. The TAPS *Institute of Hope and Healing*, in partnership with the Hospice Foundation of America, provides on-site and web-based professional training to supplement TAPS internal training programs. Training focuses on the effective use of active listening skills, familiarity with all TAPS programs and resources, identifying suicide risk, maintaining professional and personal boundaries, confidentiality, self-care, and when to make referrals to professional mental health providers.

Having lived through their own military loss experiences, TAPS peer mentors intimately understand military tragedies and survivors' unique needs [41]. Peer mentors thus serve as role models and "beacons of hope" to newly bereaved survivors during this phase of grief recovery. Peer mentors are trained to listen without judging, empathizing with the bereaved, and sharing similar experiences as appropriate in order to help them find validation, normalization, and hope for the future. With the help of peer mentors, the survivor is encouraged to shift focus from the death of his or her loved one to remembering the life that was lived and to do the hard work of reorganizing family systems and roles.

Hopeful reappraisal is also facilitated through TAPS *Health and Wellness* programs. These activities take place over several days in nature-based locations and are designed to bring together small groups of survivors to further build a sense of community, again capitalizing on peer support. TAPS *Health and Wellness* events include physical activities such as kayaking, hiking, skiing, mountain climbing, and horseback riding. Time is also reserved for conversation and reflection throughout the program. Activities are designed to encourage survivors to get out of their comfort zones, face challenges in nature, share their experiences with other survivors, form relationships, experience a sense of belonging, and learn new methods and strategies for coping with grief.

TAPS Togethers provide similar opportunities for survivors to assemble and support one another by sharing common experiences. These are 1-day programs held across the country that bring survivors together in an organized social setting and guided by TAPS peer mentors. Examples of *TAPS Togethers* include coffee shop gatherings, museum trips, local community baseball games, horse riding camps, outdoor adventures, yoga classes, potluck dinners, and community service projects.

For children, the hopeful reappraisal phase likewise includes opportunities to work through the loss and envision a hopeful future. Children have access to a supportive and nurturing social environment, which can help them process the trauma they have experienced and work through the emotions they may not be able to express while at home. At TAPS *Good Grief Camps*, children are paired with members of the military who have volunteered to serve as *military mentors* for the duration of the program. Engagement in these programs facilitates a sense of community among child survivors and an awareness that the military organization continues to honor the life and legacy of their fallen loved ones. Activities include group sessions to teach healthy coping skills including age-appropriate ways of communicating and expressing their emotions around grief.

Positive Integration

The focus in the third phase is to help survivors develop a positive sense of meaning from their loss and integrate it into their life patterns while looking ahead to a positive future. This aligns with Worden's task of adjusting to a new world without the deceased and reintegrating into the social world without the lost loved one [44].

Military survivors often differ from nonmilitary survivors in how they view and interact with the world, and may be uniquely situated to experience post-traumatic growth (PTG) following a traumatic loss. For example, they are more familiar with frequent major life disruptions such as military moves and deployment separations [46]. For the bereaved, post-traumatic growth (PTG) can be understood as positive personal changes that result from the survivor's struggles to deal with trauma and its psychological consequences. Survivors will continue to experience grief and will likely have times of escalated sensitivity around anniversaries of their loss, but the emotions surrounding the loss may be less severe.

Many survivors in this phase work to transform the pain of grief into personally meaningful, pro-social activities. TAPS peer mentors and the entire TAPS community of survivors continue to serve as important peer support elements and role models facilitating healthy grief recovery. Survivors are also encouraged to take advantage of resources and educational materials available through the TAPS *Institute of Hope and Healing.*

For children, the third phase is primarily about reintegration – how to go on with a life in which their loved one, usually a father or mother, is gone, while accepting the feelings of loss this entails. Survivors in this phase will eventually shift away from a focus on grief and death to one of honoring their loved one's life while going on with their own.

TAPS *Sports and Entertainment* programs offer additional opportunities to shift grief into a positive frame. These programs provide families and loved ones of the fallen opportunities to connect with their favorite sports teams to honor the life and legacy of their fallen military members. For example, several major sports teams have partnered with TAPS to bring grieving children to meet with their favorite players. Sports and Entertainment programs span multiple generations with special events for kids and opportunities for grieving adults to share the stories of how their loved ones enjoyed their favorite sports teams and players. Survivors from all types of losses and all relationships to the fallen are able to come together in a positive environment where they can connect with other military survivors and learn they are not alone in their grief.

While empirical studies of TAPS programs are somewhat limited, there is now extensive evidence that peer support-based programs like TAPS are effective in facilitating healthy recovery for people experiencing a range of mental health challenges [15, 26, 43]. One study that looked at a subgroup of military survivors who used TAPS programs found that survivors who had a greater number of contacts with TAPS showed higher levels of posttraumatic growth and resilience [46]. The same study also determined that bereaved survivors who had a higher number of engagements with TAPS tended to have lower levels of depression, anxiety, and suicidal ideation. Interestingly, among the survey respondents, those who also had served as peer mentors showed even higher levels of PTG and resilience. These results suggest that survivors who go on to assist other survivors derive increased benefits and growth from their experiences.

All TAPS programs are structured around the model of peer-based emotional support and follow recognized best practices that have been identified in this domain [47]. This peer-based approach provides accessible, nonthreatening, and free services that work to decrease the survivor's sense of isolation and build a feeling of hope for a positive future, thereby facilitating healthy adaptation to loss.

Since 1994, TAPS has been providing critical support for grieving survivors of a military death and is a valuable resource for military healthcare providers. TAPS has assisted thousands of survivors who have experienced a military death. In 2018 alone, over 19,000 phone calls were fielded by the TAPS 24/7 Military

Survivor Hotline and over 30,000 hours spent by TAPS peers talking with newly bereaved survivors. Over 14,000 military survivors made contact with TAPS in 2018 through some one of its programs, to include over 400 grief seminars, TAPS Togethers, Sports and Entertainment engagements, Health and Wellness programs, or camps held across the country.

In the next and final section, we provide some evidence-based suggestions on what constitutes a successful and effective peer support program for bereaved survivors.

Key Ingredients of Successful Peer Support Programs for the Bereaved

What are the essential elements in a peer support program for the bereaved? The following recommendations are based on a review of the literature and a survey of experts with experience leading peer support programs for bereaved [47]. Several quotes are also taken from this work in order to help illustrate some of the points below.

Easily Accessible and Responsive Regardless of the mechanism for providing support (whether crisis response teams, hotlines, face-to-face, or some other mode), peer support services for the bereaved must be easily accessible around the clock and on weekends. Death can strike at any time, and a survivor may reach out for help at any hour of the day or night. When the call comes, it is important that peer support be available and responsive. Peer support programs must be able to respond quickly with appropriate help when the need arises.

Confidentiality Bereaved persons seeking peer support place a high value on confidentiality. Most of them don't want to see their personal circumstances, feelings, and reactions to become public information. Thus, it is essential that the program has procedures in place to insure that privacy is maintained, and the bereaved need to be reassured of this. A police psychologist involved in peer support programs described this issue as follows:

Well, confidentiality is very, very important. One of the reasons there is a mistrust of mental health professionals among police officers is that they are going to go back to the organization and tell the story about you. That is something that turned off a lot of officers toward external programs such as EAPs (Employee Assistance Programs).

Once you lose trust, your program is going to go down the toilet. And I've seen it happen in other departments. You get a peer supporter who starts talking in small talk with some other officer, and, 'Hey, you know John Jones down there, we just had him in here. He's a drunk. You know he's got depression' or something like that. The next thing you know, nobody comes in anymore! So keep quiet. It's private - it should be a private conversation. It should stay that way.

Provide a Safe Environment In peer support programs, it is important to provide a "safe environment," a place where the bereaved feels welcomed and respected and free of judgment. This includes the physical environment in face-to-face support situations, as well as the social-emotional environment which is primarily established by the peer supporter. The ability of the peer supporter to "just listen" contributes to an atmosphere of safety and respect. In part, the creation of a safe environment includes reassuring the bereaved survivor that the peer support relationship is not short-term, but can continue into the future. Confidentiality is also an important element here.

Matching of Peer Supporter to the Bereaved It is important to find the closest possible match between the peer supporter and the person receiving the support. The more similarities between the peer supporter and the person receiving support, the more quickly they will form a connection of trust and openness. The most important aspect of this match concerns the nature of the loss experience. For example, if the bereaved experienced a death by suicide, it is best if the peer supporter has also experienced a death by suicide. A father who has lost a child has greater commonality of experience with other bereaved fathers, as compared to bereaved mothers.

Beyond cause of death and relationship to the deceased, the bereaved will more readily relate to and trust a peer supporter who has likewise lived and worked in the same occupational environment as them, as, for example, police, firefighters, or military personnel. On this point, one peer support program manager said:

> Peer supporters have their own experiences, so they know how to relate, and that's what you've got to have. Because a (survivor), whether it's a soldier, a marine, a cop, a fireman, is not going to talk to a stranger. Period. Because they haven't been there. They haven't walked the walk.

Thus, in addition to the shared experience of loss, it is important that the peer supporter has a good understanding of the occupational culture and context of the bereaved. Many aspects of the job culture are implicit and can be assumed when the peer supporter comes from the same occupational culture. This applies also to family members, whether spouses, parents, or children in many circumstances. For example, military spouses share a broad experience of the military lifestyle and culture, which helps in forming a social bond with a newly bereaved military widow.

Careful Selection of Peer Supporters In selecting people to serve as peer supporters, it's important to choose individuals who have successfully worked through their own loss and who are not presently dealing with unresolved grief issues or other life problems. Also, peer supporters should have good self-awareness and understand their own motivations for volunteering. A desire to serve is also an important consideration in selecting peer supporters.

Some peer support organizations have developed guidelines or rules of thumb to assist in the selection of peer supporters for the bereaved. For example, the TAPS program requires that peer supporters be at least 18 months past their own loss experience. When working with volunteers, it's also important to recognize that some people who volunteer may simply not be suited for the kind of work that peer supporters do and should not be selected. Desired qualities in a peer supporter are discussed further below.

Partnership with Professional Mental Healthcare Providers Another critical consideration in formulating an effective peer support program for bereaved concerns the need for professional clinical staff members who can step in and assist a survivor – or the peer supporter – when the situation calls for it. Peer supporters for the bereaved should have quick and easy access to clinical staff to consult and advise on difficult cases. It's also a good idea to have a protocol in place for assessing suicide risk in the bereaved and the potential need for a mental health referral. Clinical staff members should be available for consultation and also to guide peer supporters on setting proper boundaries in terms of what kinds of assistance to give to survivors and when to seek help from professional clinicians.

Training of Peer Supporters Peer support programs for the bereaved must invest the necessary time and resources to appropriately train their peer supporters. The type of training and content will vary to some degree across programs, but some core training is essential. For example, it's important that peer supporters have a good understanding of the culture they are working with, whether that's police, military, or some other group. Training for peer supporters should also include developing tools to use when supporting another to include active listening skills, emotional interviewing, guidance on how to assess risk levels in clients, self-care, and knowing when and how to seek professional guidance and support.

Knowing when to seek clinical help also involves staying alert to boundaries, the ability to recognize and maintain appropriate roles. Ongoing or refresher training is also valuable for peer supporters working with bereaved. This is important not only for maintaining critical skills but also provides a means of monitoring the mental health, compassion fatigue, and well-being of peer supporters. According to one expert:

> Really good training on what are appropriate boundaries and basic skills is incredibly important. And then monitoring and support and education along the way, because peer support, especially with a population like suicide loss where they often have trauma and mental health issues. Regular check-ins, monitoring, education are really important so they (peer supporters) don't burn out or become overwhelmed.

Monitoring and Care of Peer Supporters Serving as a peer supporter to those who have experienced a sudden or traumatic death is a difficult work and can be emotionally exhausting and lead to burnout to include compassion fatigue. There are a number of ways that peer supporters can receive support in their work, including from staff and other peer supporters. Peer supporters should also receive training on how to monitor themselves and to recognize when they should ask for help. The program should have systems in place for monitoring the peer supporters and providing assistance and guidance when needed. Regular meetings or debriefing sessions with peer supporters and staff can be an excellent way of monitoring peer supporters and identifying when some individuals may need rest or assistance. As one peer support expert described it:

> We know that we can say to our teammates, 'you know what? I need a break. I need to go take a nap, I need to go for a walk. I can't talk to this person right now. I'm filled up.' So we become each other's real strong support system. … It's an understanding that this is difficult work, it's complex, and it can be exhausting and there might be times when you need to take a break.

Another important element of support for the peer supporters as described by Castellano (2012) is "resilience, affirmation and praise" [22]. This primarily refers to the praise and reinforcement peer supporters give to bereaved for their progress and positive accomplishments. This also applies to peer supporters who benefit from receiving recognition and positive feedback from their superiors and peers for their good work. This feedback reinforces the sense of meaning and importance for peer supporters, while also serving to enhance their resilience.

Desirable Qualities in a Peer Supporter

Qualities needed in a peer supporter for the bereaved fall into five key categories. The peer supporter should (1) have closely similar experience (to the bereaved); (2) be a good communicator; (3) be authentic and trustworthy; (4) have good judgment – be aware of boundaries – and (5) have a calm, agreeable disposition. These qualities are further discussed below.

Closely Similar Experience This means first of all that the peer supporter should have a similar background or experience to the person being assisted. The peer supporter thus is able to draw on this shared life experience in order to form a rapid connection to the bereaved. The peer supporter should also be someone who has successfully coped with or recovered from whatever the difficult experience was and so is able to provide an inspirational role model and living example that adversity can be overcome.

Having similar shared experiences facilitates rapid formation of a strong connection between peer supporter and bereaved. The bereaved is provided with an immediate role model of someone who has experienced the same, or similar devastating loss, and is coping with their loss in a positive manner. This eases communication and also instills hope for a more positive future.

Good Communicator Good communication skills are perhaps an obvious essential quality for peer supporters. In large part, this involves an ability *to listen* and focus completely on the person being supported. Along with listening, peer supporters should show empathy, compassion, and a sense of humor and be attuned to body language in communications. These qualities allow the peer supporter to establish a connection with the bereaved and help to create an environment in which the survivor feels safe in revealing highly sensitive thoughts and feelings.

Finally, part of being a good communicator for peer supporters means being nonjudgmental, to refrain from imposing one's own views and interpretations on the bereaved. They should allow the bereaved to progress at their own pace and not try to overly direct the process. Every individual is different, and there can be no rigid formula to fit everyone. The peer supporter must be careful to be nonjudgmental and always an attentive listener.

Authentic and Trustworthy Ideally, peer supporters for the bereaved are motivated by a sincere desire to help others who have experienced a loss, as opposed to seeking some personal gain. The peer supporter should be successfully coping with her/his own loss and have the maturity and wisdom to put the needs of the survivor to the forefront. When the peer supporter is authentically motivated to assist the survivor, he or she is more quickly seen as someone who can be trusted and relied upon. This contributes also to the bereaved person's sense of being in a "safe environment" with the peer supporter.

Authenticity in this sense is believed to be a key contributor to building up the survivor's sense of trust in the peer supporter. This makes good theoretical sense. As described by Rotter (1971) nearly 50 years ago, trust is the generalized expectancy that the other person is (1) honest; (2) unselfish, not going to take advantage of me; and (3) reliable, or "knows his stuff" [48]. The authentic and trustworthy peer supporter is thus one who is honest, unselfish, and knowledgeable.

Good Judgment: Aware of Boundaries Good judgment involves the awareness of one's own limitations, strengths and weaknesses, and sound knowledge and judgment about boundaries in providing peer support. Peer supporters need to exercise good judgment as to when and how much to talk about themselves (self-disclosure) when assisting a bereaved survivor.

As mentioned earlier, the peer supporter must recognize the limits of his or her role and be willing and able to step back and seek help from a clinical professional when needed. This calls for a certain level of modesty in the peer supporter and a realistic understanding of his/her own capabilities.

Calm, Agreeable A final desirable quality in peer supporters for the bereaved is a calm and agreeable disposition. Peer supporters should project a calm, assured manner, and a desire to help, without being judgmental in any way of the bereaved. Along with this, it is helpful if the peer supporter can maintain a steady and pleasant speaking voice, avoiding rushed and/or harsh tones.

Internet-Based Peer Support for the Bereaved

Recent years have seen an increase in online support and discussion forums for people experiencing various difficulties, including grief following the death of a loved one. Given the ease of access and convenience, this trend is likely to grow. What is the evidence that peer support via the Internet is effective in facilitating healthy coping with grief?

While the research is somewhat limited, a recent review of studies in this area concluded that Internet-based approaches are generally helpful to the bereaved, though not as effective as face-to-face modalities [34]. Five out of six studies reviewed demonstrated benefits to users, including lower depression and symptoms of grief. For example, a study in Finland looked at bereaved mothers who posted messages to an online grief discussion forum [49]. The researchers found that posted messages were both giving and receiving emotional and practical support. Mothers reported feeling accepted into a group of others with similar experiences and that they benefited from their participation.

Another study in this area compared suicide survivors receiving Internet-based peer support with those receiving face-to-face support in peer groups of survivors [50]. While both groups showed significant reductions in grief symptoms, the face-to-face participants were lower, notably in depression and suicidal thinking. Participants also reported that the Internet forum was easy to access and convenient, for example, being available late at night without having to leave home. Some users also reported that they preferred the online forum over family and friends, whose responses were often dismissive and not helpful.

In yet another study of Internet-based peer support, bereaved suicide survivors involved in an Internet only support group in the Netherlands showed decreased levels of depression and increased well-being over a 12-month period [31]. An interesting study along these lines examined oncology nurses who were regularly exposed to dying patients on their jobs. Nurses participated in a "virtual world" peer support activity over a 10-week period [51]. Using a 3-D multiuser virtual environment known as "Second Life" (www.secondlife.com/destinations/learning), nurses logged in to a private meeting space and as avatars participated in group discussions and storytelling sessions regarding their job-related requirements. The group sessions were facilitated and moderated by an experienced grief counselor. Results showed that nurses who participated had an increased sense of meaning in their work, improved well-being, and reduced feelings of isolation. In addition to the convenience and enhanced privacy offered by this Internet-based approach, the authors suggest that the greater realism generated by the virtual world framework and use of avatars creates a deeper engagement and sense of presence for participants, thus enhancing the experience. This Internet-based approach may prove to be more beneficial than simple chat groups or online forums. More research is clearly needed on various Internet-based peer support activities for the bereaved to determine what the most effective methods are and when and for whom.

Conclusion

Peer support programs in various forms are growing in popularity and are used increasingly to assist bereaved individuals who have been affected by death. While not a replacement for definitive clinical care in more severe cases, peer support programs can be highly beneficial to those suffering grief after a loss and may in fact prevent many complicated grief reactions from ever developing. This chapter has reviewed the available research on peer support for bereaved and provided some evidence-based guidelines for what makes a successful peer support program. While situations and requirements certainly differ, these elements merit careful consideration by providers involved in developing or implementing peer support programs for the bereaved.

References

1. American Psychiatric Association. The diagnostic and statistical manual of mental disorders: DSM 5. Arlington: American Psychiatric Association; 2013.
2. Fujisawa D, Miyashita M, Nakajima S, Ito M, Kato M, Kim Y. Prevalence and determinants of complicated grief in general population. J Affect Disord. 2010;127:352–8.
3. Kersting A, Brähler E, Glaesmer H, Wagner B. Prevalence of complicated grief in a representative population-based sample. J Affect Disord. 2011;131:339–43.
4. Newson RS, Boelen PA, Hek K, Hofman A, Tiemeier H. The prevalence and characteristics of complicated grief in older adults. J Affect Disord. 2011;132:231–8.
5. Goldsmith B, Morrison RS, Vanderwerker LC, Prigerson HG. Elevated rates of prolonged grief disorder in African Americans. Death Stud. 2008;32:352–65.
6. Ott CH, Lueger RJ, Kelber ST, Prigerson HG. Spousal bereavement in older adults: common, resilient, and chronic grief with defining characteristics. J Nerv Ment Dis. 2007;195:332–41.
7. Piper WE, Ogrodniczuk JS, Azim HF, Weideman R. Prevalence of loss and complicated grief among psychiatric outpatients. Psychiatr Serv. 2001;52:1069–74.
8. Prigerson HG, Maciejewski PK, Reynolds CF, Bierhals AJ, Newsom JT, Fasiczka A, et al. Inventory of complicated grief: a scale to measure maladaptive symptoms of loss. Psychiatry Res. 1995;59:65–79.
9. Kochanek KD, Murphy SL, Xu J, Arias E. Deaths: final data for 2017 [Internet]. National Vital Statistics Reports. 2019 [cited 2019 Nov 18]. p. 1–77. Available from: https://www.cdc.gov/nchs/data/nvsr/nvsr68/nvsr68_09-508.pdf.

10. Cozza SJ, Fisher JE, Zhou J, Harrington-LaMorie J, La Flair L, Fullerton CS, et al. Bereaved military dependent spouses and children: those left behind in a decade of war (2001–2011). Mil Med. 2017;182:e1684–90.
11. Currier JM, Holland JM, Neimeyer RA. Sense-making, grief, and the experience of violent loss: toward a mediational model. Death Stud. 2006;30:403–28.
12. Sanders CM. Risk factors in bereavement outcome. J Soc Issues. 1988;44:97–111.
13. Goldstrom ID, Campbell J, Rogers JA, Lambert DB, Blacklow B, Henderson MJ, et al. National estimates for mental health mutual support groups, self-help organizations, and consumer-operated services. Admin Pol Ment Health. 2006;33:92–102.
14. Mead S, Hilton D, Curtis L. Peer support: a theoretical perspective. Psychiatr Rehabil J. 2001;25:134–41.
15. Solomon P. Peer support/peer provided services underlying processes, benefits, and critical ingredients. Psychiatr Rehabil J. 2004;27:392–401.
16. Landers GM, Zhou M. An analysis of relationships among peer support, psychiatric hospitalization, and crisis stabilization. Community Ment Health J. 2011;47:106–12.
17. House JS. Work stress and social support. Reading: Addison-Wesley; 1981.
18. Reblin M, Uchino BN. Social and emotional support and its implication for health. Curr Opin Psychiatry. 2008;21:201–5.
19. Grauwiler P, Barocas B, Mills LG. Police peer support programs: current knowledge and practice. Int J Emerg Ment Health. 2008;10:27–38.
20. Stretch RH. Psychosocial readjustment of Canadian Vietnam veterans. J Consult Clin Psychol. 1991;59:188–9.
21. Bartone PT. Hardiness as a resiliency factor for United States forces in the Gulf War. In: Posttraumatic stress intervention: challenges, issues, and perspectives. Springfield: Charles C. Thomas; 2000. p. 115–33.
22. Castellano C. Reciprocal peer support (rps): a decade of not so random acts of kindness. Int J Emerg Ment Health. 2012;14:137–42.
23. Christensen A, Jacobson NS. Who (or what) can do psychotherapy: the status and challenge of nonprofessional therapies. Psychol Sci. 1994;5:8–14.
24. Gould RA, Clum GA. A meta-analysis of self-help treatment approaches. Clin Psychol Rev. 1993;13:169–86.
25. Solomon P, Draine J. The state of knowledge of the effectiveness of consumer provided services. Psychiatr Rehabil J. 2001;25:20–7.
26. Davidson L, Chinman M, Kloos B, Weingarten R, Stayner D, Tebes JK. Peer support among individuals with severe mental illness: a review of the evidence. Clin Psychol Sci Pract. 1999;6:165–87.
27. Chinman M, George P, Dougherty RH, Daniels AS, Ghose SS, Swift A, et al. Peer support services for individuals with serious mental illnesses: assessing the evidence. Psychiatr Serv. 2014;65:429–41.

28. Feigelman W, Jordan JR, McIntosh JL, Feigelman B. Devastating losses: how parents cope with the death of a child to suicide or drugs. New York: Springer; 2012.
29. Harrington-LaMorie J, Ruocco K. The tragedy assistance program for survivors (TAPS). In: Grief after suicide: understanding the consequences and caring for the survivors. New York: Routledge; 2011. p. 403–11.
30. Aho AL, Tarkka MT, Åstedt-Kurki P, Sorvari L, Kaunonen M. Evaluating a bereavement follow-up intervention for grieving fathers and their experiences of support after the death of a child-a pilot study. Death Stud. 2011;35:879–904.
31. Kramer J, Boon B, Schotanus-Dijkstra M, Van Ballegooijen W, Kerkhof A, Van Der Poel A. The mental health of visitors of web-based support forums for bereaved by suicide. Crisis. 2015;36(1):38–45.
32. Barlow CA, Jeannette WS, Chugh U, Rawlinson D, Hides E, Leith J. An evaluation of a suicide bereavement peer support program. Death Stud. 2010;34:915–30.
33. Feigelman W, Jordan JR, Gorman BS. Parental grief after a child's drug death compared to other death causes: investigating a greatly neglected bereavement population. Omega J Death Dying. 2011;63:291–316.
34. Bartone PT, Bartone JV, Violanti JM, Gileno ZM. Peer support services for bereaved survivors: a systematic review. OMEGA J Death Dying. 2019;80(1):137–66.
35. Kaunonen M, Tarkka MT, Paunonen M, Laippala P. Grief and social support after the death of a spouse. J Adv Nurs. 1999;30:1304–11.
36. Worden JW, Silverman PS. Grief and depression in newly widowed parents with school-age children. OMEGA J Death Dying. 1993;27:251–61.
37. Riley LP, LaMontagne LL, Hepworth JT, Murphy BA. Parental grief responses and personal growth following the death of a child. Death Stud. 2007;31:277–99.
38. Cohen E. Bereavement during the adolescent to young adult transition: a developmental resilience model. Retrieved 12 Oct 2019 from Proquest Digital Dissertations (AAT 3172770); 2005.
39. Jordan JR, McIntosh JL. Grief after suicide: understanding the consequences and caring for the survivors. New York: Routledge; 2011.
40. Feigelman W, Jordan J, Gorman B. Personal growth after a suicide loss: cross-sectional findings suggest growth after loss may be associated with better mental health among survivors. Omega J Death Dying. 2009;59:181–202.
41. Carroll B, Hudson L, Ruby D. Complicated grief in the military. In: Doka KJ, editor. Living with grief after sudden loss: suicide, homicide, accident, heart attack, stroke. London: Routledge; 1996. p. 73–88.
42. Dooley CM, Carroll B, Fry LE, Seamon-Lahiff G, Bartone PT. A model for supporting grief recovery following traumatic loss: the tragedy assistance program for survivors (TAPS). Mil Med. 2019;184:166–70.

43. Davidson L, Bellamy C, Guy K, Miller R. Peer support among persons with severe mental illnesses: a review of evidence and experience. World Psychiatry. 2012;11:123–8.
44. Worden JW. Grief counseling and grief therapy. In: Grief counseling and grief therapy. 4th ed. New York: Springer; 2009.
45. Carroll B. Survivors helping survivors heal [Internet]. Tragedy assistance program for survivors. 2019 [cited 2019 Nov 17]. Available from: https://www.taps.org/peermentors.
46. Moore M, Palmer J, Cerel J. Growth and hope after loss: how TAPS facilitates posttraumatic growth in those grieving military deaths. In: TAPS National Military Suicide Seminar. Tampa, Florida; 2018.
47. Bartone PT, Bartone JV, Gileno Z, Violanti JM. Exploration into best practices in peer support for bereaved survivors. Death Stud. 2018;42(9):555–68.
48. Rotter JB. Generalized expectancies for interpersonal trust. Am Psychol. 1971;26:443–52.
49. Aho AL, Paavilainen E, Kaunonen M. Mothers' experiences of peer support via an Internet discussion forum after the death of a child. Scand J Caring Sci. 2012;26(3):417–26.
50. Feigelman W, Gorman BS, Chastain Beal K, Jordan JR. Internet support groups for suicide survivors: a new mode for gaining bereavement assistance. Omega J Death Dying. 2008;57:217–43.
51. Rice KL, Bennett MJ, Billingsley L. Using second life to facilitate peer storytelling for grieving oncology nurses. Ochsner J. 2014;14(4):551–62.

Peer Support for Adolescents with Chronic Illness

5

Yalinie Kulandaivelu and Sara Ahola Kohut

Adolescence is a complex period of development when youth go through significant changes biologically (puberty, sexual maturation), psychologically (developing the ability to reason and think abstractly), emotionally (learning to cope with stress, manage emotions, identity development) and socially (shifting their focus from the family to their peer groups, peer influence peaks, developing intimate relationships and/or sexual relationships) in life, as they transition to adulthood [1]. It is also the period when positive health behaviours (e.g. healthy eating and exercise) are consolidated and when risky behaviours such as smoking, alcohol and

---

Y. Kulandaivelu
Institute of Health Policy, Management and Evaluation, University of Toronto, Toronto, ON, USA

Child Health Evaluative Sciences, SickKids Research Institute, Toronto, ON, USA
e-mail: yalinie.kulandaivelu@sickkids.ca

S. A. Kohut (✉)
Child Health Evaluative Sciences, SickKids Research Institute, Toronto, ON, USA

IBD Centre, The Hospital for Sick Children, Toronto, ON, Canada

Department of Psychiatry, University of Toronto, Toronto, ON, Canada
e-mail: sara.aholakohut@sickkids.ca

drug use and sexual practice first emerge and are established [1]. As such, adolescence is an important timepoint for prevention efforts [1].

Peer groups serve as reference points for adolescents who are developing their sense of identity. Identifying with peers facilitates adolescents' development of moral judgement and values and helps them determine what distinguishes them from their own parents [2]. Peer influence is most intense during adolescence, and peers may serve as important sources of information about the world outside of their family. Adolescents also spend more time with their peers and value their peers' expectations and opinions. Friends often become increasingly similar due to the power of peer influence and the propensity of adolescents to develop friendships with similar individuals in terms of background, tastes, values and interests. Adolescents and young adults with strong social skills tend to demonstrate better academic, social and emotional outcomes than those with poorer social skills [3]. Moreover, positive peer relationships during adolescence are linked to positive psychosocial adjustment in adulthood and beyond [4].

In healthcare, peer support encompasses three main types of support: informational (e.g. advice, suggestions and facts relevant to what the peer is dealing with), emotional (e.g. expressions of caring, empathy and reassurance) and appraisal (e.g. affirmation of one's feelings and behaviours, encouraging persistence to resolve problems and reassuring them that frustrations can be handled) [5]. Peer support is varied in structure, content and delivery. These relationships last anywhere from a single interaction to several years; in one-to-one or group formats; involving contact daily, weekly or monthly; and involving structured (e.g. participate in specific activities, answer specific questions, motivational interviewing) or unstructured content (e.g. discussing any choice of topics). Peer support may be delivered via a range of mediums including, but not limited to, in-person meetings, online video calling, phone calls, text messages, email, discussion forums and social media platforms. This level of variety reflects the different needs and preferences of individuals as well as the opportunities for individuals to engage in peer support activities. Peer interventions, particularly for health promotion, may involve leveraging peers' existing memberships in social networks and relationships (informal) or may involve creating these relationships and networks formally with the aim of promoting health-related goals. Finally, a key distinction to be made is between peer interventions which aim to involve adolescents with shared characteristics and experiences and those which involve a peer mentor or educator, who may or may not be trained.

Peer Support for Health Promotion

In the context of health promotion, peer support includes peer education, which is defined as "teaching or sharing of information, values and behaviours between individuals with shared characteristics such as behaviour, experience, status or social and cultural backgrounds" [6]. Peer education may be delivered by same age or older peers in formal and informal settings, including community centres, street settings, nightclubs, school classrooms or youth programs, and may occur as part of the natural communication within the social groups [7]. The underlying notion of peer education is that adolescents and young adults may learn from each other. Peers have greater credibility among young people, have shared characteristics, can act as positive role models who reinforce behavioural messages and have greater understanding and empathy for the unique context and health behaviour of young people [7]. Meta-analysis of interventions for risk behaviours such as substance use and risky sexual behaviour has identified that effective interventions take into account the social and contextual factors of the populations. Peer education and support are approaches that allow for this tailoring to occur [8]. In this context, peer interventions for adolescents have been employed for a number of different purposes, including health promotion (healthy eating, physical activity, sexual health) and prevention (conflict resolution, violence, drug use, sexually transmitted infection) [5, 7].

Peer support is particularly helpful in health promotion during adolescence as it capitalizes on peer influence during a sensitive period in social development [7]. Based on social cognitive theory, people tend to imitate the behaviour of individuals they see as similar to themselves in terms of age, appearance and life experiences/circumstances [9–11]. Peers act as role models whose successes are attainable; therefore they are perceived as realistic figures for self-comparison [9]. Support from these peers and the modelling of their behaviour thus increases motivation and persistence in positive health behaviours for adolescents. Furthermore, support offered by peer mentors or educators can be provided through schools, thereby increasing access to helping adolescents develop decision-making and problem-solving skills as well as overcome personal and social barriers to health behaviour change [12]. This peer influence is important for health promotion as it supports positive behaviour change to improve health and prevent further disease. Peer support is particularly critical in populations where youth may not have access to, or are distrustful of, health professionals (e.g. youth with mental health concerns, youth with HIV, youth in sexual and gender minority groups), as peers are credible and trusted sources of health information [7, 13–15]. Peer mentoring, whereby the individual providing support is trained, may be ideally suited to these communities as it supports access to services, supports building trust and can strengthen social networks within the community [9, 12].

Impact of Peer Interventions for Health Promotion

A number of studies have evaluated the impact of peer interventions for health promotion and have demonstrated promising improvements in health and health-related outcomes [12, 16–19]. These findings have been demonstrated across several aspects of health (e.g. smoking, sexually transmitted infections, substance use prevention, healthy eating promotion) and for knowledge, attitude and behaviour-related outcomes. In the United Kingdom, when compared to a fact-based smoking education program, youth receiving a 10-week peer mentoring program to support smoking abstinence were significantly less likely to smoke at 1-year follow-up (as measured by saliva samples) [20]. Similarly, a peer mentorship program for HIV/AIDS prevention among orphaned adolescents in southern Uganda found that participants in the program demonstrated significantly higher scores in HIV/AIDS-related knowledge, beliefs and prevention attitudes compared to non-participants in the program [15]. A quasi-experimental study examined the impact of a 6-week peer education intervention for improving sugar-sweetened beverage intake for adolescents in Canada; peer education delivered by multiple peer educators resulted in a significant decrease in sugar-sweetened beverage intake at 3-month follow-up [21]. While most peer interventions for health promotion vary in delivery, length and format, longer program lengths may demonstrate greater improvements in health or health-related outcomes. A randomized controlled trial evaluating a year-long peer mentoring program to prevent substance use in youth with an HIV/AIDS-positive parent compared to a wait-list control group found that youth in the intervention arm had significantly lower rates of drug use. This study identified a dose effect, as the number of peer mentoring sessions attended was correlated with reduced substance use [22]. While a number of studies demonstrate improvements in health or health-related outcomes, the evidence for long-term impact continues to grow as studies with long-term follow-ups and longer interventions are conducted. Overall, there is a strong evidence that suggests peer interventions are effective in a wide variety of contexts.

Peer interventions are effective and appropriate upstream interventions for promoting healthy eating, physical activity and sexual health and reducing smoking, substance use and other risk behaviours to prevent development of chronic illness. These interventions benefit from being adapted to their specific goals and contexts as well as demonstrate a dose effect. Peer support interventions are also effective in promoting the health of adolescents who have already been diagnosed with chronic illnesses.

Peer Support for Chronic Illnesses

For adolescents with chronic illness, the process of gaining independence from their parents and furthering friendships with their peers is often disrupted by illness management (e.g. symptom management, attending medical appointments and procedures) [23]. At a time in development when becoming part of a peer group becomes an important aspect of an adolescent's life, the need to manage a chronic illness can disrupt attempts to gain peer acceptance. Adolescents with chronic illness are often isolated from their peers and have few opportunities to meet peers with the same condition. At a time when a sense of belonging to a peer group is sought, adolescents with chronic illness often lack this feeling of belonging and may experience negative effects on their social and psychological development and functioning. Studies among adolescents with chronic illnesses have demonstrated that they may have more submissive behaviours, fewer friends, lower social competence, and have reduced emotional adjustment. Adolescents with chronic illnesses have also been shown to be perceived as isolated and less likeable than their peers who havenot been diagnosed with a chronic illness [24–30]. These findings suggest that when youth who are diagnosed with chronic illnesses are less engaged in friendships and peer activities, there may also be less opportunities for them to develop and practice social skills [31]. Adults with chronic illness report significant difficulties with social interactions and isolation; thus a lack of peer support and quality friendships in adolescence may have negative outcomes that persist into adulthood.

Adolescents with chronic illness experience the added challenge of achieving self-sufficiency in illness management. Thus, formalizing peer support for adolescents with chronic illness should aim to improve health outcomes by not only targeting feelings of isolation and introducing positive role models but also in facilitating ways of learning about and practicing illness self-management skills. This is in line with the expressed needs of adolescents with chronic illness, including a need for more illness-specific knowledge, self-management strategies and meaningful social support [32–41]. Adolescents with chronic illness also report that peers may possess unique perspectives and information that healthcare providers may not be able to provide [42, 43].

Impact of Peer Interventions for Chronic Illness

Peer interventions for adolescents with chronic illness have been examined for a number of chronic conditions in a variety of formats. Many of the studies evaluating peer support for adolescents with chronic illness demonstrate positive impacts on illness-related knowledge, quality of life, attitudes towards illness, adherence to treatment plans, retention in care, school attendance and social isolation [31]. Research has shown that peer support interventions can reduce loneliness and increase social acceptance, self-efficacy and social confidence in adolescents with chronic illness. Improvements in social outcomes have been shown in online mentoring programs for adolescents with cerebral palsy or spina bifida as well as youth with diabetes or end-stage renal disease attending camp [44]. Adolescents reported that peer support put their illnesses into perspective, they felt more understood by peers than by family and friends, and they received comfort from not having to hide their medication, devices or equipment from others [40, 43]. Evidence for improvements in quality of life (QoL) in the context of peer mentoring is variable; however, some studies have demonstrated positive impacts. In a study evaluating a telephone, social media and face-to-face peer support for adolescents with type 1 or type 2 diabetes, participants in the intervention group had slight improvements in QoL and diabetes-related emotions as compared to control groups [45]. Significant improvements in HRQoL were also identified in three studies of peer-led interventions for adolescents with asthma [46]. Peer interventions may also be effective in improving chronic illness self-management. A pilot RCT of an online peer mentoring program for adolescents with JIA found significant improvements in self-management scores among intervention group participants compared to the wait-list control participants [47]. A pre-post study evaluating a peer support camp for adolescents with spina bifida demonstrated significant increases in spina bifida-related self-management activities [48]. In a mixed methods study of a peer-led camp program for adolescents with end-stage renal disease, adolescents reported increased perseverance, self-efficacy and knowledge of self-management behaviours [43]. Evidence for peer interventions improving self-management may indicate that peer support may be an effective component to include in transitional care programs from paediatric to adult healthcare. One ongoing study examines the impact of peer mentors in a transitional care program for adolescents with chronic illness [38]. Despite promising findings in illness self-management, self-efficacy and social outcomes, few studies have demonstrated the positive impacts of peer support programs in physical health outcomes. In one study examining peer support and problem-solving training for adolescents with type 1 diabetes, girls had a significant decrease in HbA1c at 12 months and a general trend towards decreased HbA1c at 24 months [49]. The evidence for impact of peer support interventions on physical health is currently limited, likely due to short follow-up periods of studies, limited measurement of physical outcomes and the difficulty of determining the intervention effect among the number of factors influencing health [7, 31]. To ensure intervention effectiveness, several issues should be considered in developing and implementing peer interventions.

Implementing Peer Interventions

Peer support programs offer flexibility in structure, delivery, length and content. However, this flexibility can result in challenges to implement these programs in real-life contexts. Below are some considerations and recommendations for developing and implementing peer support programs, including assessing for adolescent preferences, ongoing evaluation, matching peers, mode of delivery and use of peer mentors.

Assessing Adolescents' Preferences for Peer Support

An essential step in developing and implementing peer support interventions is assessing adolescents' preferences and requirements for the program. Identifying and incorporating these preferences is important in ensuring adolescents are engaged with the program and may ensure that the program meets the unique needs of this population. Peer interventions that demonstrate low to no impact on health behaviours frequently tend not to incorporate needs assessments of the target populations' preferences around what would be important to them in an intervention [50, 51]. Ongoing opportunities for adolescents to provide feedback and preferences for programming may be an option to ensure peer interventions adapt to adolescents' changing circumstances. For example, youth advisory boards have demonstrated success in supporting the development and implementation of peer support programs via ongoing feedback in samples of youth at risk of HIV as well as in samples diagnosed with inflammatory bowel disease, kidney disease, hypertension, lupus or juvenile idiopathic arthritis [14, 38]. Needs assessment studies of adolescents' preferences for peer interventions demonstrate a great deal of variation with respect to duration, frequency and length of programs, communication format (e.g. text messages, discussion forum), one-to-one or group formats and level of involvement. This suggests that peer support programs may benefit from offering individualized or flexible approaches to implementation. However, adolescents generally seem to prefer long-term relationships, with older peers, flexible options for participating and the option to meet peers in person where possible [42, 52–54]. Nevertheless, social media and other Internet-based methods of communication may be acceptable to adolescents, particularly those with mobility limitations or those residing in rural areas [41, 42, 54].

Formative Evaluation

Along with assessing adolescent preferences for peer support, formative evaluations of interventions can ensure the program works as it was intended to and to obtain preliminary feedback from participants. In one instance, a qualitative evaluation of an online peer support program for adolescents with end-stage renal disease identified issues faced by peer mentors (e.g. difficulties moderating real-time chats) and challenges with maintaining engagement among adolescents [52]. In a peer-delivered sexual health education intervention for adolescents, process evaluation revealed that adolescents preferred education to be delivered in single-gender groups instead of mixed-gender classes [55]. Formative evaluation may also aid in adapting interventions to different contexts and for unexpected needs of the youth.

Matching Mentors and Adolescents

Given the importance of peers in adolescent development, peer support programs would benefit from being mindful of how the peers are matched in a one-on-one setting or arranged together in group settings. Matching of adolescents with peer educators or mentors often varies, with some interventions grouping them by gender, personality or condition (for chronic illness). However, in practice, adolescents have found that connecting with peers is easier when they have shared interests and can reach common ground [52]. For chronic illness, qualitative evidence suggests that adolescents may prefer peer mentors who have more lived experience with their condition, are older and share similar experiences and interests [42, 52, 56]. These characteristics may take precedence over others, such as gender or personality [42].

Mode of Delivery

Previous studies suggest that adolescents may prefer peer interventions involving in-person contact with peers or peer educators

5 Peer Support for Adolescents with Chronic Illness

and mentors. However, in-person interventions involving physical activities may be challenging for adolescents with diverse mobility needs. Furthermore, they may face difficulties engaging larger numbers of youth due to location and time constraints. Interventions involving brief intensive sessions (e.g. camp interventions) may also be problematic as they cannot provide the longer-term support often requested by youth with chronic illness. For example, a study of a camp found that the social inclusion domain of HRQoL questionnaires decreased after the intervention, which the authors attributed to over identification with the group [43]. Similar findings have been reported in other camp intervention studies with adolescents with chronic illness. Likewise, peer interventions may need to exercise caution when leveraging existing social networks for intervention delivery. In one peer cannabis use intervention, substance use was mainly reduced in students who had a low level of use to begin with, while substance use increased among others [57]. In another study targeting smoking, alcohol, marijuana and cocaine use, youth who began with pro-smoking attitudes and a high proportion of friends who used tobacco tended to report higher levels of smoking after the intervention [58]. Similarly, a study evaluating a weekly peer support intervention among low-income, minority adolescents with asthma found no significant improvement in adherence to inhaled corticosteroids; in fact, they found a decrease in adherence [50]. In each of these studies, the interventions made use of existing, informal social networks among peers, instead of creating new formal networks or peer mentors. Thus, it may be the case that youth in the interventions would have risked social isolation if they had rejected group norms and reduced their smoking. MacArthur and colleagues (2016) suggest that taking account of peer norms and peer influences in existing friend groups and social networks is needed to appropriately target prevention messages and education to higher-risk groups [59]. Furthermore, there is some evidence that involving peer mentors may be more effective than peer support alone [50].

Delivery of peer interventions over the Internet or via digital mediums carries several advantages, including greater accessibility, flexibility and reach over geographic regions. Further, since so many adolescents typically connect with one another via the Internet or other digital mediums, limited additional efforts are necessary [52]. The Internet offers a variety of ways for connecting, including discussion forums; live chatting; social media networks; video calling; sharing of videos, images and text over feed-based platforms; and microblogging. The opportunity for synchronous and asynchronous communication allows for greater flexibility and for peer relationships to adapt to changing school, work and personal schedules. When planning and delivering peer interventions for delivery via digital platforms, privacy and monitoring of the interactions should be taken into account. Few mainstream digital platforms have been used for peer interventions due to limited control over privacy, as well as feasibility challenges of monitoring relationships between mentors/educators and adolescents. However, many of the studies conducted using digital platforms were completed prior to 2016, and since then, features and privacy options of social media and communication platforms have developed and improved features such as end-to-end encryption, multiple authentication, verification and personalized privacy settings. As digital platforms for peer interventions become more common, program developers may need to consider how engagement with the intervention may influence the benefits to adolescents. For example, in a study evaluating a discussion forum with live chat options for adolescents with chronic kidney disease, the authors reported that some adolescents did not actively post on the discussion forum, indicating different doses and benefits from the program for participants [52].

Involvement of Peer Mentors/Educators

Peer interventions for adolescent health can involve adolescents with shared characteristics or illness, or they can include peer mentors facilitating these groups and/or providing one-to-one support. In the chronic illness context, peer mentors tend to be older and have more lived experience with their condition. This aligns with reported preferences of youth with chronic illness when seeking peer support [42, 52, 56]. When considering the use of peer mentors versus peer support, it is important to consider how to train mentors and the potential impacts of mentorship on the mentor's own well-being.

Training for Peer Mentors/Educators

Most studies of peer interventions involve some form of training for peer mentors or educators. Training usually involves brief in-person or online sessions or modules where training content is provided by healthcare providers or study teams [31]. In one case, current peer mentors trained future peer mentors for the program. While there is currently no consensus on the optimal amount of training necessary for peer interventions provided in group settings, training in classroom or group management may be useful to peer educators or mentors and ultimately influence the success of the programs [6, 54]. Training peer mentors in groups is ideal as it provides an opportunity to create a peer group among the mentors. Furthermore, while training may occur at the start of the intervention, regular opportunities for communication may be beneficial to peer mentors to discuss challenges as they arise. These opportunities can help peer educators and mentors to consolidate skills, share strategies that work and those that do not and provide peer support to one another [6, 60]. For example, in a camp intervention for adolescents with end-stage renal disease, mentors ("buddies") had daily check-ins with other mentors and supervisors to discuss any issues that required attention [43]. In some cases, peers are trained using approaches from counselling that tend to be more formal and similar to standard teaching methods. This additional level of training may impact how peers interact with adolescents and require more ongoing training support and supervision. Thus, it is essential for peer support and peer mentorship programs to consider their goals and how formal or informal the peer intervention aims to be [51].

Impact on Peer Mentors/Educators

A number of qualitative and survey-based studies report positive impacts on peers' knowledge, skills and personal development [6]. However, studies of peer interventions have seldom completed rigorous quantitative evaluations on the impact of programs on peer mentors or educators or their experience in the intervention [6]. One RCT study examined health-related quality of life (HRQoL) of peer mentors in a camp-based peer intervention for adolescents with end-stage renal disease; the authors reported a significant improvement in the independence domain of HRQoL after participation in the camp [43]. A qualitative study of young adult peer mentors living with juvenile idiopathic arthritis or chronic pain condition found that peer mentors benefited from the social connection with fellow mentors as well as their mentees. They felt a sense of pride in their role in their mentee's growth and experienced personal growth as a result of being a mentor [61]. When planning evaluations and research study designs of peer interventions, the impact on peer educators and mentors should also be included in the design.

Conclusion

Peer support is ideally suited to adolescents due to the importance of peers in adolescents' development and the number of changes adolescents go through during this sensitive period of development. For adolescents with chronic illness, engaging with peers is complicated by the burden of managing a chronic illness. Thus, there is a need for delivering and adapting peer support interventions to align them with the ways adolescents currently interact with one another (e.g. technology, social media). When developing peer interventions, "peers" should be defined as those who are similar to the target audience in terms of experiences, ethnicity, gender identity, socioeconomic status and interests; peer mentors should be slightly older; and for chronic illness they should have the illness themselves (or an illness with similar symptom profile). Matching of adolescents with peers should occur based on expressed preferences of adolescents and prioritizing adolescents' preferences in design of the program and emphasizing flexibility. If peer mentors are included in the intervention, training is essential to ensure intervention effectiveness and that peer mentors are supported. Finally, some evidence suggests that the inclusion of trained peer mentors in interventions may be more effective than peer support alone.

References

1. Williams PG, Holmbeck GN, Greenley RN. Adolescent health psychology. J Consult Clin Psychol. 2002;70:828.
2. Bishop AJ, Inderbitzen MH. Peer acceptance and friendship: an investigation of their relation to self-esteem. J Early Adolesc. 1995;15(4):476–89.
3. Brown BB, Larson J. Peer relationships in adolescence. In: Handbook of adolescent psychology. New York: Wiley; 2009.
4. Bagwell CL, Newcomb AF, Bukowski WM, Bagwell CL, Newcomb AF, Bukowski WM. Preadolescent friendship and peer rejection as predictors of adult adjustment. Child Dev. 1998;69(1):140–53.
5. Dennis CL. Peer support within a health care context: a concept analysis. Int J Nurs Stud. 2003;40:321–32.
6. Strange V. Peer education. In: MacDowall W, Bonnell C, Davies M, editors. Health promotion practice. Berkshire: Open University Press; 2006. p. 97–111.
7. Parkin S, McKeganey N. The rise and rise of peer education approaches. Drugs Educ Prev Policy. 2000;7(3):293–310.
8. Kirby D, Obasi A, Laris BA. The effectiveness of sex education and HIV education interventions in schools in developing countries. World Health Organ Tech Rep Ser. 2006;938:103.
9. McAlister AL, Perry CL, Parcel GS. How individuals, environments, and health behaviors interact: Social cognitive theory. In Glanz K, Rimer BK, Viswanath K (Eds.), Health behavior and health education: Theory, research, and practice. Jossey-Bass. 2008;169–88.
10. Simons R, Conger R, Whitbeck L. A multistage social learning model of the influences of family and peers upon adolescent substance abuse. J Drug Issues. 1988;18(3):293–315.
11. Bandura A. Social cognitive theory of self-regulation. Organ Behav Hum Decis Process. 1991;50:248–87.
12. Petosa RL, Smith LH. Peer mentoring for health behavior change: a systematic review. Am J Health Educ. 2014;45(6):351–7.

13. Sheffield JK, Fiorenza E, Sofronoff K. Adolescents' willingness to seek psychological help: promoting and preventing factors. J Youth Adolesc. 2004;33(6):495–507.
14. Swendeman D, Arnold EM, Harris D, Fournier J, Comulada WS, Reback C, et al. Text-messaging, online peer support group, and coaching strategies to optimize the HIV prevention continuum for youth: protocol for a randomized controlled trial. J Med Internet Res. 2019;8:e11165.
15. Nabunya P, Ssewamala FM, Mukasa MN, Byansi W, Nattabi J. Peer mentorship program on HIV/AIDS knowledge, beliefs, and prevention attitudes among orphaned adolescents: an evidence based practice. Vulnerable Child Youth Stud [Internet]. 2015;10(4):345–56. Available from: https://doi.org/10.1080/17450128.2015.1115157.
16. Yip C, Gates M, Gates A, Hanning RM. Peer-led nutrition education programs for school-aged youth: a systematic review of the literature. Health Educ Res. 2016;31:82–97.
17. Maticka-Tyndale E, Barnett JP. Peer-led interventions to reduce HIV risk of youth: a review. Eval Program Plann. 2010;33:98–112.
18. MacArthur GJ, Harrison S, Caldwell DM, Hickman M, Campbell S, ORCID: http://orcid.org/0000-0002-7966-0700, Hickman M, ORCID: http://orcid.org/0000-0001-9864-459X RAI-O http://orcid.org/Hariso, Georgie JM, et al. Peer-led interventions to prevent tobacco, alcohol and/or drug use among young people aged 11–21 years: a systematic review and meta-analysis. Albrecht Armstrong, Borenstein, Borenstein, Botvin, Botvin, Campbell, Dishion, Eckhardt, Elder, Ellickson, Ellickson, Ellickson, Faggiano, Foxcroft, Foxcroft, Fromme, Fuller, Gates, Guyatt, Harden, Harden, Higgins, Ioannidis, Kelly, Kim, Kincaid, Klepp, A, editor. Addiction [Internet]. 2016;111(3):391–407. Available from: http://ovidsp.ovid.com/ovidweb.cgi?T=JS&PAGE=reference&D=emed17&NEWS=N&AN=616593099.
19. Rose-Clarke K, Bentley A, Marston C, Prost A, et al. Peer-facilitated community-based interventions for adolescent health in low- and middle-income countries: a systematic review. PLoS One [Internet]. 2019;14(1):e0210468. Available from: https://journals.plos.org/plosone/article/file?id=10.1371/journal.pone.0210468&type=printable.
20. Campbell R, Starkey F, Holliday J, Audrey S, Bloor M, Parry-Langdon N, et al. An informal school-based peer-led intervention for smoking prevention in adolescence (ASSIST): a cluster randomised trial. Lancet. 2008;371(9624):1595–602.
21. Lo E, Coles R, Humbert ML, Polowski J, Henry CJ, Whiting SJ. Beverage intake improvement by high school students in Saskatchewan, Canada. Nutr Res. 2008;28(3):144–50.
22. Rosenblum A, Magura S, Fong C, Curry P, Norwood C, Casella D. Effects of peer mentoring on HIV-affected Youths' substance use risk and association with substance using friends. J Soc Serv Res. 2006;32:45–60.

23. Wysocki T, Hough BS, Ward KM, Green LB. Diabetes mellitus in the transition to adulthood: adjustment, self-care, and health status. J Dev Behav Pediatr. 1992;13:194–201.
24. Forgeron PA, King S, Stinson JN, McGrath PJ, MacDonald AJ, Chambers CT. Social functioning and peer relationships in children and adolescents with chronic pain: a systematic review. Pain Res Manag. 2010;15(1):27–41.
25. Engström I. Mental health and psychological functioning in children and adolescents with inflammatory bowel disease: a comparison with children having other chronic illnesses and with healthy children. J Child Psychol Psychiatry. 1992;33(3):563–82.
26. Cortina S, McGraw K, de Alarcon A, Ahrens A, Rothenberg ME, Drotar D. Psychological functioning of children and adolescents with eosinophil-associated gastrointestinal disorders. Child Health Care. 2010;39(4):266–78.
27. LeBovidge JS, Lavigne JV, Donenberg GR, Miller ML. Psychological adjustment of children and adolescents with chronic arthritis: a meta-analytic review. J Pediatr Psychol. 2003;28(1):29–39.
28. Noll RB, Vannatta K, Koontz K, Kalinyak K, Bukowski WM, Davies WH. Peer relationships and emotional well-being of youngsters with sickle cell disease. Child Dev. 1996;67(2):423–36.
29. Trzepacz AM, Vannatta K, Davies WH, Stehbens JA, Noll RB. Social, emotional, and behavioral functioning of children with hemophilia. J Dev Behav Pediatr. 2003;24(4):225–32.
30. Warner EL, Kent EE, Trevino KM, Parsons HM, Zebrack BJ, Kirchhoff AC. Social well-being among adolescents and young adults with cancer: a systematic review. Cancer. 2016;122(7):1029–37.
31. Kohut SA, Stinson J, van Wyk M, Giosa L, Luca S. Systematic review of peer support interventions for adolescents with chronic illness. Int J Child Adolesc Health. 2014;7:183.
32. Lehmkuhl HD, Merlo LJ, Devine K, Gaines J, Storch EA, Silverstein JH, et al. Perceptions of type 1 diabetes among affected youth and their peers. J Clin Psychol Med Settings. 2009;16(3):209–15.
33. Stinson JN, Toomey PC, Stevens BJ, Kagan S, Duffy CM, Huber A, et al. Asking the experts: exploring the self-management needs of adolescents with arthritis. Arthritis Care Res. 2008;59(1):65–72.
34. Mackner LM, Ruff JM, Vannatta K. Focus groups for developing a peer mentoring program to improve self-management in pediatric inflammatory bowel disease. J Pediatr Gastroenterol Nutr. 2014;59(4):487–92.
35. Stinson JN, Sung L, Gupta A, White ME, Jibb LA, Dettmer E, et al. Disease self-management needs of adolescents with cancer: perspectives of adolescents with cancer and their parents and healthcare providers. J Cancer Surviv. 2012;6(3):278–86.

36. Kulandaivelu Y, Lalloo C, Ward R, Zempsky WT, Kirby-Allen M, Breakey V, et al. Exploring the needs of adolescents with sickle cell disease to inform a digital self-management and transitional care program: a qualitative study. JMIR Pediatr Parent. 2018;1:e11058.
37. Breakey VR, Bouskill V, Nguyen C, Luca S, Stinson JN, Kohut SA. Online peer-to-peer mentoring support for youth with hemophilia: qualitative needs assessment. JMIR Pediatr Parent. 2018;1(2):e10958.
38. Wiemann CM, Graham SC, Garland BH, Hergenroeder AC, Raphael JL, Sanchez-Fournier BE, et al. Development of a group-based, peer-mentor intervention to promote disease self-management skills among youth with chronic medical conditions. J Pediatr Nurs [Internet]. 2019;48:1–9. Available from: https://doi.org/10.1016/j.pedn.2019.05.013.
39. Hughes J, Wood E, Smith G. Exploring kidney patients experiences of receiving individual peer support. Health Expect. 2009;12(4):396–406.
40. Bergeron S, Noskoff K, Hayakawa J, Frediani J. Empowering adolescents and young adults to support, lead, and thrive: development and validation of an AYA Oncology Child Life Program. J Pediatr Nurs [Internet]. 2019;47:1–6. Available from: https://doi.org/10.1016/j.pedn.2019.04.001.
41. Lu Y, Pyatak EA, Peters AL, Wood JR, Kipke M, Cohen M, et al. Patient perspectives on peer mentoring: type 1 diabetes management in adolescents and young adults. Diabetes Educ. 2015;41(1):59–68.
42. Ahola Kohut S, LeBlanc C, O'Leary K, McPherson AC, Jelen A, McCarthy E, Nguyen C, Stinson J. Peer mentoring needs and wants of youth with chronic conditions: a qualitative analysis. Child Care Health Dev. 2019. Status: Manuscript under review.
43. Sattoe JN, Jedeloo S, Van Staa A. Effective peer-to-peer support for young people with end-stage renal disease: a mixed methods evaluation of Camp COOL. BMC Nephrol. 2013;14(1):1–14.
44. Stewart M, Barnfather A, Magill-Evans J, Ray L, Letourneau NN. Brief report: an online support intervention: perceptions of adolescents with physical disabilities. J Adolesc. 2011;34:795–800.
45. Lim PK, Cheng TS, Hui YCA, Lim STJ, Lek N, Yap F, et al. D-buddy peer support for better health outcomes in adolescents with diabetes mellitus. Int J Pediatr Endocrinol [Internet]. 2015;2015(S1):P15. Available from: http://www.ijpeonline.com/content/2015/S1/P15.
46. Kew KM, Carr R, Crossingham I. Lay-led and peer support interventions for adolescents with asthma. Cochrane Database Syst Rev. 2017;2017(4).
47. Stinson J, Ahola Kohut S, Forgeron P, Amaria K, Bell M, Kaufman M, et al. The iPeer2Peer program: a pilot randomized controlled trial in adolescents with juvenile idiopathic arthritis. Pediatr Rheumatol [Internet]. 2016;14(1):1–10. Available from: https://doi.org/10.1186/s12969-016-0108-2.
48. O'Mahar K, Holmbeck GN, Jandasek B, Zukerman J. A camp-based intervention targeting independence among individuals with spina bifida. J Pediatr Psychol. 2010;35:848–56.

49. Løding R, Wold J, Skavhaug Å, Graue M. Evaluation of peer-group support and problem-solving training in the treatment of adolescents with type 1 diabetes. Eur Diabetes Nurs. 2007;4(1):28–33.
50. Mosnaim G, Li H, Martin M, Richardson DJ, Belice PJ, Avery E, et al. The impact of peer support and mp3 messaging on adherence to inhaled corticosteroids in minority adolescents with asthma: a randomized, controlled trial. J Allergy Clin Immunol Pract [Internet]. 2013;1(5):485–93. Available from: https://doi.org/10.1016/j.jaip.2013.06.010.
51. Harden A, Weston R, Oakley A. A review of the effectiveness and appropriateness of peer-delivered health promotion interventions for young people. In: Database of Abstracts of Reviews of Effects (DARE): Quality-assessed Reviews [Internet]. Centre for Reviews and Dissemination (UK); 1999.
52. Nicholas DB, Picone G, Vigneux A, McCormick K, Mantulak A, McClure M, et al. Evaluation of an online peer support network for adolescents with chronic kidney disease. J Technol Hum Serv. 2009;27(1):23–33.
53. Kohut SA, Stinson JN, Ruskin D, Forgeron P, Harris L, Van Wyk M, et al. iPeer2Peer program: a pilot feasibility study in adolescents with chronic pain. Pain. 2016;157:1146–55.
54. Masuda JR, Anderson S, Letourneau N, Sloan Morgan V, Stewart M. Reconciling preferences and constraints in online peer support for youth with asthma and allergies. Health Promot Pract. 2013;14(5):741–50.
55. Strange V, Oakley A, Forrest S. Mixed-sex or single-sex sex education: how would young people like their sex education and why? Gend Educ. 2003;15:201–14.
56. Cassano J, Nagel K, O'Mara L. Talking with others who "just know": perceptions of adolescents with cancer who participate in a teen group. J Pediatr Oncol Nurs. 2008;25(4):193–9.
57. Ellickson PL, Bell RM. Drug prevention in junior high: a multi-site longitudinal test. Science. 1990;247(4948):1299–305.
58. Valente T, Ritt-Olson A, Stacy A, Unger J, Okamoto J, Sussman S. Peer acceleration: effects of a social network tailored substance abuse prevention program among high-risk adolescents. Addiction. 2007;102(11):1804–15.
59. MacArthur GJ, Harrison S, Caldwell D, Hickman M, Campbell R. Peer-led interventions to prevent tobacco, alcohol and/or drug use among young people aged 11–21 years: a systematic review and meta-analysis. Addiction. 2016;111(3):391–407.
60. Morisky DE, Nguyen C, Ang A, Tiglao TV. HIV/AIDS prevention among the male population: results of a peer education program for taxicab and tricycle drivers in the Philippines. Health Educ Behav. 2005;32(1):57–68.
61. Ahola Kohut S, Stinson J, Forgeron P, Luca S, Harris L. Been there, done that: the experience of acting as a young adult mentor to adolescents living with chronic illness. J Pediatr Psychol Special Issue Adolesc Young Adult Health. 2017;42(9):962–9.

Peer Support for Older Adults

6

Kimberly A. Van Orden and Julie Lutz

Introduction

People around the world are living longer, and the number of older adults is increasing—a phenomenon termed "population aging." According to US Census Bureau projections, the worldwide population of older adults (those who are 65 years old or older) is projected to reach 1.5 billion by 2050, underscoring the importance of promoting healthy (or "successful") aging. One means of promoting healthy aging is drawing upon strengths of older adults. Studies from the gerontological literature have demonstrated that later life is not typically a time of isolation and despair: despite losses in function, cognitive capacity, and social network size, rates of depression decline in later life [1]. In fact, emotional well-being frequently *increases* with age, as evidenced by negative emotions being experienced less often (e.g., anger), and the ability to manage and change one's emotions (i.e., emotion

---

K. A. Van Orden (✉) · J. Lutz
Department of Psychiatry, University of Rochester School of Medicine & Dentistry, Rochester, NY, USA
e-mail: Kimberly_vanorden@urmc.rochester.edu

regulation) often improves with age, in part due to increased motivation to experience positive emotions and accumulated life experiences that allow older adults to make effective choices regarding situations to approach or avoid [1]. Some research suggests that loneliness actually decreases as we grow older [2]. Research from lifespan developmental theorists has described the best approach to healthy aging as involving an increased focus on the most meaningful aspects of life—typically relationships—rather than a focus on losses or death. Of course, some older adults do struggle with the transitions of later life and do become isolated and depressed, and thus a focus on promoting positive meaningful social relationships should be beneficial to those who struggle as well.

Promoting supportive, meaningful relationships as a means to support healthy aging is a commonplace practice in many communities. However, these programs are rarely integrated into medical care and often do not reach many older adults who could benefit, in part because most programs have not been rigorously tested. Peer support interventions for older adults vary considerably in terms of objectives, mode of delivery, whether monetary compensation is provided for the individual providing support, and what is provided—friendship, instrumental support, support for managing health conditions, or mentoring for behavior change. How "peer" is defined also varies significantly across programs and studies. In this chapter, we provide an overview of three broad categories of peer support programs available for older adults—peer companionship, peer specialists, and patient navigation—based on our analysis of the literature on peer support in older adults. Figure 6.1 provides a graphical overview of our framework. These categories are based on the definition of "peer" and therefore the function the peer provides in the intervention. For peer companionship programs, peers are older adults who do not provide a formal intervention, but instead build a relationship with a "care receiver" (or patient/client) for the purposes of support, companionship, and friendship. Peer specialist programs involve matching individuals with a shared experience or medical condition for the purpose of providing education or intervention—thus peer in this instance means someone with the same

Peer companionship

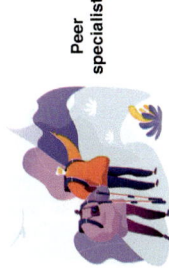

Objectives: Reduce loneliness & isolation; help an older adult remain independent in the community by providing instrumental support or to providing respite for caregivers.

Definition of peer: older adult (no matching on medical conditions, etc.).

Program content: fostering a supportive, meaningful relationship.

Example program: The Senior Companions Program of the Senior Corps (part of the Corporation for National and Community Service): https://www.nationalservice.gov/programs/senior-corps/senior-corps-programs/senior-companions

Resources for learning more:
- National Council on Aging webinar on "Fostering Peer Support to Address Behavioral Health Needs Among Older Adults," available at: https://www.ncoa.org/resources/webinar-fostering-peer-support-to-address-behavioral-health-needs-among-older-adults/
- AARP Foundation's Connect2Affect: https://connect2affect.org/
- National Association of Area Agencies on Aging: https://www.n4a.org/

Patient navigation

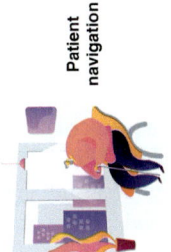

Objectives: Promote full engagement in healthcare and self-management for chronic conditions.

Definition of peer: Patient navigation programs are not always delivered by peers, but when they are, peers are individuals who have been diagnosed with the condition that is the focus of the program (e.g., cancer or diabetes).

Program content: Health information, assistance navigating appointments, care transitions, and understanding treatment information; patient activation and promotion of self-management; bridge to healthcare team to promote trust and engagement and reduce healthcare disparities.

Example program: Community Health Advisor Program at The University of Alabama at Birmingham (Patient Care Connect Program): https://www.uab.edu/onealcancercenter/outreach/community-health-advisor-program

Resources for learning more:
- National Academy of Medicine Workshop Proceedings on "Establishing Effective Patient Navigation Programs in Oncology" available at: https://www.nap.edu/download/25073#
- For social determinants of health: https://healthleadsusa.org/

Peer specialist

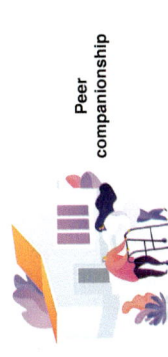

Objectives: Promote engagement in treatment for health conditions, including through increased self-management.

Definition of peer: An individual who is in recovery from a mental health or substance use disorder (though some programs for older adults are more inclusive and focus on health more broadly).

Program content: Peer specialists can provide a range of services and supports, including peer support, encouraging self-determination, health and wellness support, illness management, and education. Services provided by mental health Certified Peer Specialists (CPSs) can be reimbursed by Medicaid in several states and peer specialists are integrated into a variety of settings and clinics within VA healthcare systems.

Example program: Certified Older Adult Peer Specialists (COAPS): http://olderadultpeerspecialists.org/

Resources for learning more:
- SAMHSA peer worker website: https://www.samhsa.gov/brss-tacs/recovery-support-tools/peers
- Veterans Health Administration Peer Specialist Toolkit: https://www.mirecc.va.gov/visn4/peer_specialist_toolkit.asp

Fig. 6.1 Types of peer support programs for older adults

health condition or experience (e.g., mental illness). Patient navigation programs are provided in healthcare settings and involve peers providing support and education regarding how to optimize healthcare supports and services. In the sections below, we describe the purpose of these programs and what they consist of generally when provided with older adults. We then describe evidence supporting effectiveness for these programs when available. Finally, we provide examples of existing programs for older adults to illustrate the range of available programs. We end by discussing the concept of "social prescribing" and ways in which these programs could be integrated more fully into medical care for older adults.

Peer Companionship

Peer companionship programs are those that provide friendship/support to older adults. There is a wide range of types of programs that can be considered peer companionship that are described as befriending, peer support, and peer companionship. These programs focus on the development of a supportive relationship and can best be characterized by what they do *not* provide: these programs do not provide education (e.g., on a medical condition) or focus on promoting behavior change (e.g., exercise). These programs may vary in the degree to which they emphasize instrumental support (e.g., daily tasks), with some programs focused on this function to help older adults live independently in the community or to provide respite to caregivers, with others focusing on developing a supportive peer relationship as the primary goal to alleviate loneliness and isolation.

Research studies examining the effectiveness of this type of intervention vary considerably in terms of targeted populations, inclusion criteria, outcome measures, duration of the intervention, and amount of training provided. Not surprisingly, the literature assessing the effectiveness of peers providing friendship/support is mixed. Few randomized trials have been conducted. A meta-analysis examining the effect of befriending on depressive symptoms (24 RCTs) found a significant effect (described as "modest") in favor of befriending [3]. Of note, this paper included programs that used volunteers *or* paid workers, including professionals, as long as the peer relationship was focused on emotional support and was non-directive. A more recent meta-analysis of befriending examined a range of patient-reported outcomes, including depression, loneliness, quality of life, self-esteem, social support, and well-being [4]. This study only included programs provided by volunteers (i.e., not paid workers or professionals). The meta-analysis with 14 studies (11 RCTs and 3 quasi-experimental) yielded a significant effect of befriending (standardized mean difference of 0.18), but only when the outcome was the primary patient-reported outcome specified for that trial (i.e., the outcomes varied across the trials included in the analysis due to differing specified primary outcomes). Results for specific outcomes across trials (i.e., irrespective of the trial's specified primary outcome—depression, social support, loneliness, quality of life) did not indicate benefit for befriending. Existing studies have not examined programs already implemented in the community. With each trial developing its own unique program, it is difficult to draw conclusions about effectiveness given that these interventions are highly complex and thus vary substantially from study to study. In order to draw generalizable conclusions, research is needed that tests existing standardized programs with implementation manuals.

One example of a peer companionship program for older adults is the "Senior Companions" program, which is part of the US nationwide program, Senior Corps, operated by the federal agency, the Corporation for National and Community Service (CNSC), which also operates other national service programs, including AmeriCorps (for younger adults). The Senior Corps is a network of national service programs for Americans 55 years and older and consists of three programs, Senior Companions, Senior Grandparents, and the Retired Senior Volunteer Program (RSVP). The goal of Senior Corps is improving lives and fostering civic engagement. Senior Corps programs operate in local communities in all 50 states, the District of Columbia, Puerto Rico, and the Virgin Islands. Senior Companion Program (SCP) volunteers help older adults maintain independence and remain in their own homes [5]. SCP volunteers provide friendly visiting, offer transportation to medical appointments, deliver groceries and prepare meals, help with simple chores like light housekeeping, and provide supportive phone calls. SCP volunteers complete an orientation, receive ongoing support and training, and may be paid a small stipend (for income-eligible volunteers) to help remove the barriers to volunteering and ensure participants do not incur additional costs while serving. Older adults who are paired with a SCP volunteer typically spend 3–4 hours per week with the SCP volunteer they are matched with and continue in the program for several years.

The CNSC commissioned an independent evaluation of the program that describes benefits to those receiving peer companionship [6] as well as benefits to the older volunteers providing peer companionship [7, 8]. Among those who have been matched with a SCP volunteer for at least 1 year, most report high satisfaction with the program because it helped them feel less lonely and more satisfied with their life and helped them take care of necessary errands and appointments and remain living in their home [6]. Typically, both the instrumental and supportive functions of peer companionship are described by clients; for example, one SCP client stated: "If I didn't have a Senior Companion, I would be really lost. When she comes to pick me up, I'm able to do all my errands and accomplish what I need to be home alone. It's a wonderful bond" [5]. However, data from the program evaluation were collected from individuals who actively sought out the SCP program, leaving unanswered the question of whether individuals who did not actively seek out the program—for example, those whose doctor recommended it—would engage with the program and demonstrate benefit. The Senior Connection (TSC) was a randomized trial of peer companionship provided by Senior Corps volunteers for older primary care patients (age 60 or older) who reported feeling lonely or like a burden on others and who did not seek out peer companionship services on their own (author KVO of the chapter was a Co-Investigator on the trial) [9]. Participants were randomized to up to 2 years of being matched with a peer volunteer who provided friendly visiting and supportive phone calls or care-as-usual with their physician. Results indicated reduced depression, anxiety, and feeling like a burden on others, as well as high satisfaction with the program, similar to results from the CNCS evaluation, despite the subjects not seeking out the program on their own [10]. One participant (an 82 year-old female) stated: "It makes me feel better, to have somebody like her. She gives me a chance to do things I couldn't do otherwise. Walks, shopping, coffee. She's just that kind of a person."

Peer Specialists

Within mental health and substance use, peer specialists may provide support for or even deliver interventions addressing a wide range of behavioral health issues [11], with certification available in most states [12]. Traditionally, peer specialists are individuals with lived experience and in recovery from a mental illness or substance use disorder [12], though within some programs, peers sometimes include any lay volunteer of a similar demographic or user of the program, with or without a history of mental illness (e.g., WRAP, as described below). Services provided by mental health certified peer specialists (CPSs) can be reimbursed by Medicaid in several states [11, 12]. Peer specialists work in a variety of settings or programs (e.g., case management, inpatient or partial hospitalization programs, psychiatric rehabilitation, residential programs, education, and advocacy) and provide a range of services (e.g., peer support, encouraging self-determination, health and wellness support, illness management, education) both individually and in groups [11]. Various mental health-related programs for older adults utilize peer specialists or peer support; we will provide a brief overview of some examples of programs that are currently implemented in the community.

The Veterans Health Administration (VHA) division of the Veterans Administration (VA), of which adults age 65 and older constitute almost half (approximately 49%) of the treated patient population [13], has recommended utilization of peer specialist services since 2003 and currently requires peer support services to some extent within certain programs and centers [14]. Peer specialists are integrated into a variety of settings and clinics within VA healthcare systems, including residential mental health programs, psychosocial rehabilitation and recovery centers, homelessness programs, outpatient PTSD treatment, and many others [14–16]. General research shows positive outcomes of peer support, such as positive change in psychiatric symptoms [17], improved housing stability [16], patient self-perceived reductions in isolation and increases in integration into the community [18], and overall positive impact on Veteran care as perceived by local recovery coordinators (often involved in hiring, training, and supervising peer specialists) [19]. However, there is minimal research on the specific effects of peer support services for mental health in older adults.

The Wellness Recovery Action Planning (WRAP) self-management program, originally developed for serious mental illness in younger adults, has been expanded to address issues outside of serious mental illness (e.g., management of chronic health problems) and is being adapted for use with older adults and utilizes peer support from other users of WRAP [20]. Components of WRAP include a wellness toolbox, a daily maintenance plan, and action plans for varying levels of stressors or crises (i.e., triggers, early warning signs, recognizing when things are getting worse, crisis, and post-crisis) [20]. Though studies have shown that participants in WRAP demonstrate significant reductions in depressive and anxiety symptoms and improved recovery [21], greater engagement in self-advocacy [22], and reduced mental health service need and utilization [23], there are not currently published studies on its outcomes among older adults specifically.

The Certified Older Adult Peer Specialists (COAPS) program utilizes CPSs to address aging-related challenges in mental health and substance use recovery [24]. Peer specialists not only undergo the required 2-week CPS training but also complete a 3-day COAPS-specific training. These specialists are adults age 50 and older who are in recovery from mental illness and/or substance use disorders and are trained in issues related to mental health and aging, including background on aging, clinical issues (e.g., depression and anxiety, substance use, trauma, suicide), and "implementation" (e.g., motivational interviewing, positive psychology, legal issues, advocacy, and working in behavioral health systems) [24]. COAPS began in Pennsylvania and has expanded to New Jersey and Massachusetts [24]. There are no published studies to date on outcomes of this program, though program evaluations and feedback by the peer specialists indicate that they, as well as the patient population, receive benefit from involvement in the program [24].

Though a variety of peer specialist programs have been implemented with older adults, little is known about the outcomes of these programs in this population. Further studies are needed to demonstrate the benefits and possible challenges of utilizing these peer resources for promoting mental health in later life. Some additional programs are currently undergoing research on development and testing, but have yet to be widely implemented outside of research studies. For example, the "Do More, Feel Better" program aims to utilize lay peer (age 60 and older) volunteers to deliver a behavioral activation intervention for treating depression in older adults at senior centers [25, 26]. Preliminary outcomes are promising, with potential clients and potential staff expressing comfort and interest in the intervention, and enrolled clients reporting high satisfaction [25, 26]. Another example is PeerTECH, a technology-based self-management intervention for older adults with serious mental illness that integrates in-person sessions led by a CPS and follow-ups throughout the intervention via text messaging and use of a smartphone app [27, 28]. Preliminary data demonstrate improvements in self-management of psychiatric symptoms and a signal for improvement in self-management of chronic health problems, quality of life, and empowerment [27, 28]. Though further formal evidence is needed for the beneficial outcomes of peer specialists and peer support programs on mental health in older adult-specific populations, these programs provide a promising avenue for enhancing interventions and reaching older adults who may not be engaged with care in traditional settings.

Patient Navigation

Patient navigation is a final category of peer-delivered interventions for older adults that we cover in this chapter. As with the other types of peer interventions, a standard, universal definition of patient navigation does not exist, complicating program evaluation and research studies. The definition used here is that patient navigation is a healthcare-focused intervention that can be delivered by a range of individuals, from nurses, to social workers, to community health workers, to peers [29]. While definitions and functions vary across programs and research studies, the core function of patient navigation is helping patients navigate the healthcare system by providing education, practical assistance in overcoming barriers to treatment, and emotional support, though other functions can be provided, including patient activation (and self-management assistance) and managing care transitions. Patient navigation was originally developed to reduce racial and socioeconomic disparities in oncology [29] and has been adapted to a range of chronic medical conditions, including diabetes, HIV, cardiovascular disease, chronic kidney disease, dementia, and comorbid chronic conditions [30].

The majority of research studies on patient navigation have been conducted in cancer with peers as navigators and phone-delivered interventions; while not all participants in these studies were older adults, given the conditions under study, many participants are age 60 and older [30]. However, with older adults, patient navigation programs may be more likely to use health professionals, such as nurses, rather than peers, at least among programs tested in research studies [31]. Studies examine a range of primary outcomes, including promoting healthcare engagement through such indicators as following through on referrals for cancer screenings and adherence to treatment, to health outcomes specific to the condition under study, as well as health-related quality of life, and mortality. Outcomes vary across these types of outcomes, with significant findings most often observed for improving healthcare engagement behaviors, with less clarity regarding findings for health outcomes and quality of life, which may be due to limitations of the research designs (such as small sample sizes) [30].

An example of a peer-delivered patient navigator program specifically designed for older patients is the Patient Care Connect Program at the University of Alabama Birmingham Health System Cancer Community Network. The program focuses on patient activation and patient empowerment and frames its objective as health promotion rather than disease management. The program includes education on health promotion including increasing exercise (in a safe manner) and managing pain and fatigue. Patient satisfaction with the program is high, with 89.5% of surveyed patients (over 1 year of program evaluation) reporting they would recommend the program to another cancer survivor [32]. Program objectives, including healthcare utilization, reduced costs, increased quality of life, and reduced symptom burden, are continuously monitored and support benefit of the program for patients and the health system, including significant cost savings accounted for, in part, by significant reductions in emergency department visits, hospitalizations, and intensive care unit admissions [33].

Future Directions

Many peer support programs for older adults are siloed within either the community or medical sectors, without strong linkages between the healthcare system and community agencies that often provide peer support or that provide services that may complement peer support by address social determinants of health. Community health workers are one type of peer support that is an exception to this because this type of program is specifically designed to build bridges between healthcare and community supports that address social determinants of health. Community health workers provide a similar function to patient navigators but are focused on providing navigation regarding linkage to community services and meeting needs regarding social determinants of health, such as lack of healthy food, safe housing, and social isolation. In the UK, where the healthcare system operates under a different financial model from the USA, community health workers can be prescribed by primary care physicians (GPs), which is a concept known as "social prescribing" [34]. Patients can thereby be referred to a range of non-medical opportunities ranging from assistance with housing to a gardening group. In the USA, this practice is less common, but enthusiasm for the practice is increasing as the importance of addressing social determinants of health becomes even clearer. Health Leads is one organization in the USA that champions addressing social determinants of health (https://healthleadsusa.org), including through community health workers. Community health worker programs will vary in the extent to which they fit the definition of peer support, as these positions are typically paid and not restricted to a certain age nor lived experience with an illness. However, many programs aim to employ individuals of similar cultural backgrounds of the individuals the programs will serve; and, by definition, these individuals are not health professionals.

Rigorous research studies supporting social prescribing are lacking, but the practice deserves serious consideration for promoting the health and well-being of older adults [35]: implementing social prescribing for older adults has the potential to increase uptake of interventions, such as peer support, for the individuals who stand to benefit most and who might not otherwise seek out such programs from community agencies. Evaluation data from the UK suggests that social prescribing is acceptable to patients and associated with high satisfaction [36]. Some have proposed innovative solutions to making social prescribing and linkage to community and peer supports feasible and accessible for older adults within the US healthcare system, including developing digital health programs to serve the functions of community health workers [37]. As the number of older adults increases worldwide without a corresponding increase in the number of geriatrics-trained health professionals, supplementing healthcare interventions with peer support has the potential to mitigate workforce challenges in a way that also builds upon a developmental strength of later life—prioritizing meaningful social relationships.

References

1. Charles ST, Carstensen LL. Social and emotional aging. Annu Rev Psychol. 2010;61:383–409.
2. Bruce LD, Wu JS, Lustig SL, Russell DW, Nemecek DA. Loneliness in the United States: a 2018 National Panel Survey of demographic, structural, cognitive, and behavioral characteristics. Am J Health Promot. 2019:890117119856551.
3. Mead N, Lester H, Chew-Graham C, Gask L, Bower P. Effects of befriending on depressive symptoms and distress: systematic review and meta-analysis. Br J Psychiatry. 2010;196(2):96–101.
4. Siette J, Cassidy M, Priebe S. Effectiveness of befriending interventions: a systematic review and meta-analysis. BMJ Open. 2017;7(4):e014304.
5. Corporation for National and Community Service. Senior companions: make independence a reality. 2020.
6. Pratt D, Lovegrove P, Birmingham C, Lombas L, Vicinanza N, Georges A, et al. Senior Companion Program independent living performance measurement survey: process, rationale, results, and recommendations. North Bethesda; 2014.
7. Georges A, Fung W, Smith J, Liang J, Sum C, Gabbard S. Longitudinal Study of Foster Grandparent and Senior Companion Programs: service delivery implications and health benefits to the volunteers. North Bethesda, MD; 2018.
8. Tan EJ, Georges A, Gabbard SM, Pratt DJ, Nerino A, Roberts AS, et al. The 2013–2014 Senior Corps Study: Foster Grandparents and Senior Companions. Public Policy & Aging Report. 2016;26(3):88–95.
9. Van Orden KA, Stone DM, Rowe J, McIntosh WL, Podgorski C, Conwell Y. The Senior Connection: design and rationale of a randomized trial of peer companionship to reduce suicide risk in later life. Contemp Clin Trials. 2013;35(1):117–26.
10. Conwell Y, Van Orden KA, Stone DS, LiKamWa McIntosh W, Messing S, Rowe J, et al. Peer companionship for mental health of older adults in primary care: a pragmatic, non-blinded, parallel group, randomized controlled trial. American Journal of Geriatric Psychiatry. 2020. https://doi.org/10.1016/j.jagp.2020.05.021.
11. Salzer MS, Schwenk E, Brusilovskiy E. Certified peer specialist roles and activities: results from a national survey. Psychiatr Serv. 2010;61(5):520–3.
12. Wolf J. National trends in peer specialist certification. Psychiatr Serv. 2018;69(10):1049.
13. Wang J, Cidade M, Larsen M, Pearman G, Schimpf M, Dhanireddy P. 2018 survey of veteran enrollees' health and use of health care. 2019.
14. Chinman M, Henze K, Sweeney P. Peer specialist toolkit: implementing peer support services in VHA. In: Center VNEMPE, Center VMPR, editors. https://www.mirecc.va.gov/visn4/peer_specialist_toolkit.asp.

15. Kumar A, Azevedo KJ, Factor A, Hailu E, Ramirez J, Lindley SE, et al. Peer support in an outpatient program for veterans with posttraumatic stress disorder: translating participant experiences into a recovery model. Psychol Serv. 2019;16(3):415–24.
16. Ellison M, Schutt R, Yuan L, Mitchell-Miland C, Glickman M, McCarthy S, et al. Impact of peer specialist services on residential stability and behavioral health status among formerly homeless veterans with cooccurring mental health and substance use conditions. Med Care. 2020;
17. Chinman M, McCarthy S, Bachrach RL, Mitchell-Miland C, Schutt RK, Ellison M. Investigating the degree of reliable change among persons assigned to receive mental health peer specialist services. Psychiatr Serv. 2018;69(12):1238–44.
18. McCarthy S, Chinman M, Mitchell-Miland C, Schutt RK, Zickmund S, Ellison ML. Peer specialists: exploring the influence of program structure on their emerging role. Psychol Serv. 2019;16(3):445–55.
19. Chinman M, Salzer M, O'Brien-Mazza D. National survey on implementation of peer specialists in the VA: implications for training and facilitation. Psychiatr Rehabil J. 2012;35(6):470–3.
20. Copeland M, Mead S. Wellness recovery action plan and peer support. Chandler: Peach Press; 2004.
21. Cook JA, Copeland ME, Floyd CB, Jonikas JA, Hamilton MM, Razzano L, et al. A randomized controlled trial of effects of Wellness Recovery Action Planning on depression, anxiety, and recovery. Psychiatr Serv. 2012;63(6):541–7.
22. Jonikas JA, Grey DD, Copeland ME, Razzano LA, Hamilton MM, Floyd CB, et al. Improving propensity for patient self-advocacy through wellness recovery action planning: results of a randomized controlled trial. Community Ment Health J. 2013;49(3):260–9.
23. Cook JA, Jonikas JA, Hamilton MM, Goldrick V, Steigman PJ, Grey DD, et al. Impact of Wellness Recovery Action Planning on service utilization and need in a randomized controlled trial. Psychiatr Rehabil J. 2013;36(4):250–7.
24. Zubritsky C, Keogh B, Cantiello H. Certified Older Adult Peer Specialist Program: a peer-based model addressing co-morbidities in older adults living in the community. Rehabilitation and Community Providers Association Conference; Hershey, 2016.
25. Raue PJ, Dawson A, Hoeft T, Russo J, Ferguson D, Green L, et al. Acceptability of a lay-delivered intervention for depression in senior centers. Aging Ment Health. 2019:1–8.
26. Raue PJ, Sirey JA, Dawson A, Berman J, Bruce ML. Lay-delivered behavioral activation for depressed senior center clients: Pilot RCT. Int J Geriatr Psychiatry. 2019;34(11):1715–23.
27. Fortuna KL, Storm M, Naslund JA, Chow P, Aschbrenner KA, Lohman MC, et al. Certified peer specialists and older adults with serious mental illness' perspectives of the impact of a peer-delivered and technology-

supported self-management intervention. J Nerv Ment Dis. 2018;206(11):875–81.
28. Fortuna KL, DiMilia PR, Lohman MC, Bruce ML, Zubritsky CD, Halaby MR, et al. Feasibility, acceptability, and preliminary effectiveness of a peer-delivered and technology supported self-management intervention for older adults with serious mental illness. Psychiatry Q. 2018;89(2):293–305.
29. National Academies of Sciences Engineering, and Medicine. Establishing effective patient navigation programs in oncology: proceedings of a workshop. Washington, DC; 2018.
30. McBrien KA, Ivers N, Barnieh L, Bailey JJ, Lorenzetti DL, Nicholas D, et al. Patient navigators for people with chronic disease: a systematic review. PLoS One. 2018;13(2):e0191980.
31. van Ee IB, Hagedoorn M, Slaets JP, Smits CH. Patient navigation and activation interventions for elderly patients with cancer: a systematic review. Eur J Cancer Care (Engl) 2017;26(2). https://pubmed.ncbi.nlm.nih.gov/27991704/.
32. Rocque GB, Partridge EE, Pisu M, Martin MY, Demark-Wahnefried W, Acemgil A, et al. The patient care connect program: transforming health care through lay navigation. J Oncol Pract. 2016;12(6):e633–42.
33. Rocque GB, Pisu M, Jackson BE, Kvale EA, Demark-Wahnefried W, Martin MY, et al. Resource use and medicare costs during lay navigation for geriatric patients with Cancer. JAMA Oncol. 2017;3(6):817–25.
34. Alderwick HAJ, Gottlieb LM, Fichtenberg CM, Adler NE. Social prescribing in the U.S. and England: emerging interventions to address patients' social needs. Am J Prev Med. 2018;54(5):715–8.
35. Hamilton-West K, Milne A, Hotham S. New horizons in supporting older people's health and wellbeing: is social prescribing a way forward? Age Ageing 2020;49(3):319–26. https://doi.org/10.1093/ageing/afaa016.
36. Woodall J, Trigwell J, Bunyan AM, Raine G, Eaton V, Davis J, et al. Understanding the effectiveness and mechanisms of a social prescribing service: a mixed method analysis. BMC Health Serv Res. 2018;18(1):604.
37. Vos J, Gerling K, Linehan C, Siriwardena AN, Windle K. Understanding care navigation by older adults with multimorbidity: mixed-methods study using social network and framework analyses. JMIR Aging. 2018;1(2):e11054.

Parent Peer Models for Families of Children with Mental Health Problems

Mary C. Acri, Emily Hamovitch, Anne Kuppinger, and Susan Burger

An estimated 1.9–6.1 million children between the ages of 3 and 17 have a diagnosable mental health condition including anxiety, depression, and oppositional defiant disorder [1]. The intractable and chronic nature of many mental health disorders, coupled with a lack of appropriate treatment and support, have a deleterious impact upon a child's educational and occupational functioning,

---

M. C. Acri (✉)
McSilver Institute for Poverty, Policy, and Research,
New York, NY, USA

Department of Child and Adolescent Psychiatry, NYU Langone School of Medicine, New York, NY, USA
e-mail: mac2281@nyu.edu

E. Hamovitch
New York University, McSilver Institute for Poverty Policy and Research, New York, NY, USA

A. Kuppinger
NYU Child Study Center/IDEAS, Department of Child and Adolescent Psychiatry, New York, NY, USA

S. Burger
Albany, NY, USA

© Springer Nature Switzerland AG 2021
J. D. Avery (ed.), *Peer Support in Medicine*,
https://doi.org/10.1007/978-3-030-58660-7_7

relationships, and physical, emotional, and behavioral health [2–4]. Child-onset mental health difficulties also have a significant impact upon the family. Alongside parenting challenges associated with their child's mental health problems, caregivers are tasked with overseeing and advocating for their child's treatment needs in a barrier-laden service system [5, 6], yet they often lack their own emotional support and information about resources, services, and information about treatment options for their child [6]. These difficulties, coupled with experiencing burden, stigma, and blame for their child's condition [5, 6], puts caregivers at high risk for stress, strain, and emotional distress [5, 7–12].

Supporting caregivers is of paramount importance for the health and wellbeing of the entire family; reduction in parental stress, for example, not only enhances the emotional health of parents but is also associated with improvements in therapeutic outcomes among youth [13]. However, the child mental health system has historically subverted caregivers' needs, and their involvement in treatment has been primarily to support the child [14]. In the 1980s, a new model of service delivery was formalized in which parent peers, defined as trained parents/primary caregivers of children with mental health needs, provided similarly situated families with an array of services such as emotional support, information about mental health and treatment, and linkages to services for the child and themselves [14]. This chapter provides an overview of parent peers and the services they provide, including the multiple theories underlying parent peer support programs, evidence supporting these models, and future directions for the field.

Qualifications and Roles

Parent peers are referred to in the literature as peer support specialists, peer and parent advocates, family peer advocates, and family or parent advisors. By definition, a parent peer has to have had lived experience as the primary caregiver for a child with a mental health problem and has navigated the child-serving system [14–17], as it is their lived experience that is believed to make them uniquely qualified to engage parents and caregivers facing similar issues [18, 19]. Additional criteria vary but may also include age and educational requirements (e.g. being 18 years of age or older and having a high school diploma), completion of trainings, holding a valid credential, and prior paid or volunteer experience working or volunteering providing peer parent support [20].

Unlike other peer models, parent peers focus on the parent/ primary caregiver and support them to take an active role in decision-making, navigating services, and developing their capacity to meet the needs of their child and family. This often occurs in collaboration with clinicians and other providers who are focused more centrally on the child's treatment needs. Within this capacity, the roles that parent peers assume are multifaceted, yet comprised primarily of providing education and information, facilitating linkages to supports, and providing emotional support, skill development, and advocacy.

By way of example, Hoagwood and colleagues [14] conducted a review and synthesis of family support programs and found that peers engage in services which include: informational/ educational support (for example, providing families with information about resources that may be available to them); instructional/ skills development (for example, coaching caregivers on effective ways to address their child's behaviors); emotional and affirmation support (promoting caregivers' feelings of being affirmed and appreciated); instrumental support (such as providing concrete services); and advocacy (such as assisting parents to understand their rights and advocate effectively for the services their child is entitled to.)

Formal training programs for these roles are beginning to emerge. Rodriguez and colleagues [21] describe the development and evaluation of a professional program to enhance parent peers' professional skills, called the Parent Empowerment Program (PEP). The PEP training was originally designed as a 5-day in-person training and currently consists of a combination of online self-learning modules followed by a two-day in-person training and a series of 12 weekly group coaching calls. PEP training fulfils the training requirement for the New York State Family Peer

Advocate Credential (FPA). Approximately 400 individuals currently hold a valid FPA Credential [22]. Evaluation of the training program provided systematically collected information about peer activities over time. It indicated that the job functions of parent peer workers include provision of information/education, advocacy, tangible assistance, and emotional support, but that emotional support and service access issues appear to be a key focus of the peer's role.

Theory

Often, reports of any peer-delivered intervention do not state an explicit theory about the mechanisms underlying how it will impact the outcomes under investigation, but rather center around a series of values, ideas, and beliefs [23]. Without an underlying theory, it is difficult to know if these mechanisms are being carried through into practice, which can lead to a lack of congruence between design, implementation, and evaluation [23]. Therefore, theories are necessary to understand how parent peer programs are intended to work, along with the expected intermediate and long-term changes in caregiver, child, and family outcomes.

A theoretical basis for understanding the potential effectiveness of peer support has been offered in the literature to a limited extent. One theory is Festinger's Social Comparison Theory. This theory postulates that individuals self-evaluate based on the comparison of their own beliefs and desires against those of another person's [24]. It proposes that individuals seek to improve their self-esteem and enhance themselves by making comparisons with others [25]. Within the context of peer support, vulnerable or at-risk individuals work with peers who have made successful changes, thereby encouraging comparison and positive behavior change [26]. Moreover, people are more likely to compare themselves to another when they perceive the person to be similar to themselves. Parent peers may be perceived by individuals to be more similar than a traditional clinician, due to their shared lived experience. This shared connection may provide common ground between the two individuals upon which to change [26].

A second theory which may provide a theoretical rationale for the value of peer support is Bandura's Social Learning Theory. This theory posits that behavior is learned from the environment through the process of observational learning [27]. In other words, desirable behaviors are modeled and the effects of these behaviors can be determined in the process of observational learning. These observed and newly learned behaviors can then serve as a guide for future action [26]. Within the context of peer support, parents have the opportunity to observe new behaviors through role modeling from a parent peer [28], which may enhance the caregiver's confidence, perceived empowerment and sense of personal agency.

Rogers' Diffusion of Innovation theory [29] has also been offered as an explanatory framework for peer support. This theory explains how an idea or new behavior gains momentum and is "adopted" by others. Adoption of new or innovative behaviors relies on the perception that they are superior to current behavior, that they align with one's values, and that there are opportunities to observe what happens when others adopt the new behaviors. Although specific to youth peers, an Australian study that aimed to identify the key features, impacts, and outcomes associated with peer-based programs draws on this theory to explain how, in a group peer program, long-standing or negative attitudes or beliefs can change through exposure to positive coping strategies adopted by credible and positive peer role models. New innovative and acceptable behaviors that were adopted in their youth peer-based program included improved help-seeking behavior, pro-social behaviors, and alternatives to risk behaviors [30].

Aside from specific theories, key components that are responsible for the positive impacts of peer support have been identified in the literature. Because of their personal experience, parent peers have credibility and are able to engender trust. Shared experiences also enable parent peers to adopt a nonjudgmental attitude [31]. In the case of parent peer programs, these trusting relationships can assist caregivers in becoming more actively engaged in their child's services [32–37]. In this same way, parent peers are often seen as authentic because they can relate to common challenges and have found their way to support their child and family to move forward in positive ways. This lived-experience helps the families be hopeful that things can get better.

Research Evidence

The diversity of roles and settings in which parent peers work is reflected in the research about these models. A synthesis of this literature identifies four main foci: (1) the feasibility and acceptability of peer programs; (2) mental health services utilization, (3) caregiver and family processes, and, (4) symptoms and functioning.

Feasibility and Acceptability

Feasibility and acceptability studies primarily test innovative models in which the program is being delivered in a new setting or the role of the peer deviates from the typical services they offer. A consensus of these studies suggests that parent peer programs are highly feasible to deliver and perceived as being acceptable from the perspectives of caregivers and peers. For example, Acri et al. developed and tested a detection and outreach model in which parent peers screened caregivers for symptoms of depression, provided information about mental health and treatment, connected at-risk caregivers to mental health services for a formal assessment, and using an evidence-informed approach, taught caregivers how to be empowered participants in their treatment. This model was tested both in freestanding family support organizations, which serve caregivers of children with emotional and behavioral problems [38, 39], and in the child welfare system [15, 40]. In both studies, results showed the intervention was highly feasible to deliver, based upon metrics including number of sessions completed, fidelity to the intervention, and attendance, and acceptable from the perspectives of parent peers and caregivers in that peers felt comfortable delivering the intervention and caregivers viewed parent peers inquiring about their mental health favorably. Moreover, Butler and Titus [16] found a preventative peer-delivered parenting intervention delivered in primary care settings for families of preschool youth at risk for behavior problems was feasible for parent peers to deliver as measured by the number of physicians who referred caregivers to peers, the number of peers who completed the training and caregiver attendance. And, January et al. [5] found that a telephone intervention for caregivers of children at risk for behavioral or emotional problems was delivered with fidelity, which is an important criterion for assessing feasibility.

Mental Health Services Utilization

Peer-delivered services also appear to facilitate treatment utilization for caregivers. For example, caregivers at risk for depression who participated in Acri et al. [38, 39] detection and outreach model and reported a strong working alliance with their parent peer were also more likely to access mental health services and reported fewer perceived barriers to help seeking (Hamovitch et al., in press). This finding is consistent with results of Radigan et al. [41] study, which surveyed over 1200 caregivers across New York State who had accessed public mental health services and found that caregivers who worked with a parent peer attended more mental health sessions for themselves than caregivers who did not utilize parent peer services, and evidenced significantly greater satisfaction with services and overall satisfaction as well.

However, the evidence isn't quite as clear for child service use. Specifically, Hoagwood et al. [14] reviewed two published studies that examined child treatment engagement: The first found the parent peer program, which aimed to facilitate treatment utilization prior to beginning Oregon's Early and Periodic Screening, Diagnosis, and Treatment Program, was associated with the child's initial engagement into treatment, but had no impact upon ongoing use of services or attendance [35]. The second study, which tested Parent Connectors, a telephone-based program for caregivers of children receiving special education and who had emotional problems, did not find any discernible impact of the peer program upon the child's utilization of treatment [42].

Caregiver and Family Processes

Studies of caregiver and familial processes also vary. Specifically, Hoagwood et al. [43] Parent Empowerment Program, which aimed to train parent peers to empower and activate caregivers to engage their children into mental health services, found no impact upon caregiver strain or empowerment, while Kutash et al. [42] Parent Connectors found significant improvements from pre- to posttest on family empowerment, but only among those who were experiencing the high levels of strain. Further, Koroloff et al. [35] found that the EPSDT pretreatment program was associated with slight improvements in the caregiver's sense of empowerment comparative to a matched comparison group. And, January et al. [5] found significant pre- to post-improvements in the caregiver's perception of social and concrete (e.g., access to supports and resources) as a result of a peer parent support program delivered by phone.

Child and Caregiver Symptoms and Functioning

A synthesis of this literature suggests that peer models are associated with multiple, positive outcomes for children and their caregivers. Results of a recent randomized controlled trial of a parent peer-delivered educational and supportive group for ethnically and racially diverse families of children with autism spectrum disorder found that caregivers in the intervention condition exhibited significant improvements in knowledge about autism and reductions in caregiver stress in comparison to caregivers receiving treatment as usual (referrals to services in the community) [44].

Additionally, studies of peer-delivered parenting programs found several improvements in child and caregiver outcomes. In comparison to a waitlist control group, for example, caregivers who received a peer-delivered parenting program evidenced significant improvements in their concerns about their child and parenting, and their children showed significant improvements in behavior, although there was no difference between this group and a waitlist control group regarding parent stress [45]. Butler and Titus [16] found a peer-delivered parenting skills intervention was associated with significant improvements in parent-reported behavior problems and parenting stress and competence from pre- to posttest, although the frequency of their preschool child's behavior problems was not significantly impacted. And, Chacko et al. [46] who examined a parent peer-delivered parenting program for families of children with ADHD found that the intervention, coupled with medication, was linked to improvements in child behavior symptoms and functioning as well as reductions in parenting stress and improved parenting behavior. However, neither Hoagwood et al. [43] nor Kutash et al. [42] found improvements in child behavior or emotional functioning due to the Parent Empowerment Program training or the Parent Connectors programs, although the primary targets for these interventions were caregiver empowerment, activation, and support, and not child emotional health or functioning.

Taken as a whole, the emerging research on parent peer models is favorable; peer-delivered interventions appear to be feasible to administer and acceptable to key stakeholders, facilitate service use by caregivers to address their own behavioral healthcare needs, increase caregiver knowledge, and improve child and caregiver emotional health and functioning. To this latter point, parenting skills programs appear to be the most effective for decreasing mental health symptoms, improving the child's functioning, reducing caregiver stress, and enhancing parenting.

Future of Peer Programs

Peer-delivered services have expanded dramatically both in the United States and globally [47]. Peer parents assume a range of roles and are embedded in a variety of settings, most states have established credentialing requirements, and parent peer delivered services are, or will soon be, a billable service under Medicaid across the United States [16, 48]. The research on parent peer models is encouraging and shows several areas of growth, including detection and outreach models for caregivers at risk (e.g., Acri et al. [38, 39]), integrated and co-located models [16, 46], and preventive programs for at-risk youth [5]. Efforts such as these illustrate the growth and promise of parent peer models for families of children with mental health difficulties.

References

1. Data and statistics on children's mental health. Retrieved from https://www.someaddress.com/full/url/.
2. Bellis MA, Lowey H, Leckenby N, et al. Adverse childhood experiences: retrospective study to determine their impact on adult health behaviors and health outcomes in a UK population. J Public Health. 2013;36:81–91.
3. Costello EJ, Angold A, Keeler GP. Adolescent outcomes of childhood disorders: the consequences of severity and impairment. J Am Acad Child Adolesc Psychiatry. 1999;38(2):121–8.
4. Washburn J, Teplin L, Voss L, et al. Psychiatric disorders among detained youths: a comparison of youths processed in juvenile court and adult criminal court. Psychiatr Serv. 2008;59:965–73.
5. January SAA, Hurley KD, Stevens AL, Kutash K, Duchnowski AJ, Pereda N. Evaluation of a community-based peer-to-peer support program for parents of at-risk youth with emotional and behavioral difficulties. J Child Fam Stud. 2016;25:836–44.
6. Shor R, Birnbaum M. Meeting unmet needs of families of persons with mental illness: evaluation of a family peer support hotline. Community Ment Health J. 2012;48:482–8.
7. Addington J, McCleery A, Addington D. Three-year outcome of family work in an early psychosis program. Schizophr Res. 2005;79:107–16.
8. Angold A, Messer SC, Stangl D, Farmer EMZ, Costello EJ, Burns BJ. Perceived parental burden and service use for child and adolescent psychiatric disorders. Am J Public Health. 1998;88:75–80.
9. Bademli K, Duman L. Effects of a family-to-family support program on the mental health and coping strategies of caregivers of adults with mental illness: a randomized controlled study. Arch Psychiatr Nurs. 2014;28:392–8.
10. Chien WT. Effectiveness of psychoeducation and mutual support group program for family caregivers of Chinese people with schizophrenia. Open Nurs J. 2008;2:28–39.
11. Dixon L, McFarlane WR, Lefley H, Lucksted A, Cohen M, Falloon I, et al. Evidence-based practices for services to families of people with psychiatric disabilities. Psychiatr Serv. 2001;52:903–10.

12. Wu P, Hoven CW, Bird HR, Moore RE, Cohen P, Alegria M, et al. Depressive and disruptive disorders and mental health service utilization in children and adolescents. J Am Acad Child Adolesc Psychiatry. 1999;38:1081–90.
13. Kazdin AE, Whitley MK. Treatment of parental stress to enhance therapeutic change among children referred for aggressive and antisocial behavior. J Consult Clin Psychol. 2003;71:504–15.
14. Hoagwood KE, Cavaleri MA, Olin SS, Burns BJ, Slaton E, Gruttadaro D, Hughes R. Family support in children's mental health: a review and synthesis. Clin Child Fam Psychol Rev. 2010;13:1–45.
15. Acri M, Hamovitch E, Gopalan G, Lalayants, M. Examining the impact of a peer-delivered program for child welfare involved caregivers upon depression and engagement in mental health services. Under Review.
16. Butler AM, Titus C. Pilot and feasibility study of a parenting intervention delivered by parent peers. Vulnerable Child Youth Stud. 2017;12:215–25.
17. Gopalan G, Lee SJ, Harris R, Acri MC, Munson M. Utilization of peers in services for youth with emotional and behavioral challenges: a scoping review. J Adolesc. 2017;55:88–115.
18. Davidson L, Bellamy C, Guy K, Miller R. Peer support among persons with severe mental illnesses: a review of evidence and experience. World Psychiatry. 2012;11:123–8.
19. Oh H, Solomon P. Role-playing as a tool for hiring, training, and supervising peer providers. J Behav Health Serv Res. 2014;41:216–29.
20. National Certified Peer Specialist (NCPS) Certification. Downloaded August 29, 2019 from https://www.mentalhealthamerica.net/national-certified-peer-specialist-ncps-certification-get-certified.
21. Rodriguez J, Olin SS, Hoagwood KE, Shen S, Burton G, Radigan M, et al. The development and evaluation of a parent empowerment program for family peer advocates. J Child Fam Stud. 2011;20:397–405.
22. Families Together in New York State (FTNYS). FPA credentialing update report; 2019.
23. Trickey H. Peer support: how do we know what works? 2016. Retrieved from https://orca.cf.ac.uk/91931/3/Trickey%20Peer%20support.pdf.
24. Festinger L. A theory of social comparison processes. Hum Relat. 1954;7:117–40.
25. Wood JV. Theory and research concerning social comparisons of personal attributes. Psychol Bull. 1989;106:231.
26. Barton J, Henderson J. Peer support and youth recovery: a brief review of the theoretical underpinnings and evidence. Can J Family Youth. 2016;8:1–17.
27. Bandura A. Observational learning. In: Donsbach W, editor. The international encyclopedia of communication. Oxford, UK: Blackwell; 2008. p. 3359–61.
28. Miller PH. Theories of developmental psychology. New York, NY: Worth Publishers; 2010.

29. Rogers EM. Diffusion of innovations: third edition. New York: The Free Press; 1983.
30. Hildebrand J, Lobo R, Hallett J, Brown G, Maycock B. My-peer toolkit: developing an online resource for planning and evaluating peer-based youth programs. Youth Stud Aust. 2002;31:53–61.
31. Mourra S, Sledge W, Sells D, Lawless M, Davidson L. Pushing, patience, and persistence: peer provider perspectives on supportive relationships. Am J Psychiatr Rehabil. 2014;17:307–28.
32. Gyamfi P, Walrath C, Burns BJ, Stephens RL, Geng Y, Stambaugh L. Family education and support services in systems of care. J Emot Behav Disord. 2010;18:14–26.
33. Hoagwood KE. Family-based services in children's mental health: a research review and synthesis. J Child Psychol Psychiatry. 2005;46:670–713.
34. Koroloff NM, Elliott DJ, Koren PE, Friesen BJ. Connecting low-income families to mental health services: the role of the family associate. J Emot Behav Disord. 1994;2:240–6.
35. Koroloff NM, Elliott DJ, Koren PE, Friesen BJ. Linking low-income families to children's mental health services: an outcome study. J Emot Behav Disord. 1996;4:2–11.
36. Osher T, Penn M, Spencer SA. Partnerships with families for family-driven systems of care. In: Stroul BA, Blau GM, editors. The system of care handbook: transforming mental health services for children, youth, and families. Baltimore: Brookes Publishing; 2008. p. 249–74.
37. Robbins V, Johnston J, Barnett H, Hobstetter W, Kutash K, Duchnowski AJ, et al. Parent to parent: a synthesis of the emerging literature. Tampa: University of South Florida, The Louis de la Parte Florida Mental Health Institute, Department of Child & Family Studies; 2008.
38. Acri MC, Frank S, Olin SS, Burton G, Ball JL, Weaver J, Hoagwood KE. Examining the feasibility and acceptability of a screening and outreach model developed for a peer workforce. J Child Fam Stud. 2015;24:341–50.
39. Acri M, Olin SS, Burton G, Herman RJ, Hoagwood KE. Innovations in the identification and referral of mothers at risk for depression: development of a peer-to-peer model. J Child Fam Stud. 2014;23:837–43.
40. Hamovitch EK, Acri M, Gopalan G. Relationships between the working alliance, engagement in services, and barriers to treatment for female caregivers with depression. Child Welfare. In Press.
41. Radigan M, Wang R, Chen Y, Xiang J. Youth and caregiver access to peer advocates and satisfaction with mental health services. Community Ment Health J. 2014;50:915–21.
42. Kutash K, Duchnowski AJ, Lynn N. School-based mental health: an empirical guide for decision-makers. Tampa: University of South Florida, Louis de la Parte Florida Mental Health Institute, Department of Child

and Family Studies, Research and Training Center for Children's Mental Health; 2006.
43. Hoagwood K, Rodriguez J, Burton G, Penn M, Olin S, Shorter P, et al. Parents as change agents: the Parent Empowerment Program for parent advisors in New York state. Paper presented at the 22nd Annual Research Conference: a system of care for children's mental health: expanding the research base, Tampa, FL; 2009.
44. Jamison JM, Fourie E, Siper PM, Trelles MP, George-Jones J, Grice AB, et al. Examining the efficacy of a family peer advocate model for Black and Hispanic caregivers of children with autism spectrum disorder. J Autism Dev Disord. 2017;47:1314–22.
45. Day C, Michelson D, Thomson S, Penney C, Draper L. Evaluation of a peer led parenting intervention for disruptive behaviour problems in children: community based randomised controlled trial. Br Med J. 2012;344:605–8.
46. Chacko A, Hopkins K, Acri M, Mendelsohn A, Dreyer B. Connecting service delivery systems to expand ADHD service provision in urban socioeconomically disadvantaged communities: a proof of concept study. Under review.
47. Repper J, Carter T. A review of the literature on peer support in mental health services. J Ment Health. 2011;20:392–411.
48. Nicholson J, Valentine A. Key informants specify core elements of peer supports for parents with serious mental illness. Front Psych. 2019;10:106–31.

# Peer Support for the Medical Community

Beverly Shin

Introduction

Healthcare workers face unique stressors in their daily encounters with illness, suffering, and death [4]. Adverse patient events such as medical error or unanticipated patient injury or death can compound providers' emotional distress and lead to poor work performance, burnout, or mental illness [51, 59, 67, 68]. Many healthcare organizations have developed robust support systems for patients and families in the event of adverse patient outcomes, but significantly fewer provide institutional support for distressed medical staff under such circumstances [8, 42]. Healthcare providers, physicians in particular, often prefer to receive support from peers rather than from employee assistance programs that have traditionally been offered to staff after medical errors or adverse events [22, 46]. As provider burnout and emotional distress in healthcare providers approach alarming levels, several institutions have established clinician peer support programs in hopes of minimizing the negative effect on patients, providers, and systems of care when adverse clinical events occur [11, 14, 21, 46, 49]. The long-

B. Shin (✉)
New York Presbyterian Hospital Weill Cornell Medicine,
New York, NY, USA
e-mail: bhs9013@nyp.org

term effectiveness of these programs remains unclear. However, the process of designing and implementing institutional peer support programs highlights salient challenges and barriers to supporting distressed clinicians after adverse patient events.

The Second Victim

Dr. Albert Wu first coined the term "second victim" in 2000 to describe the emotional distress experienced by clinical staff in the aftermath of medical errors that harm patients [65]. He identified the patient as the first victim in an adverse event and the healthcare provider as the second victim and called attention to the urgent need to support clinicians after patient safety events to prevent maladaptive responses to grief and trauma [65]. In 2009, Susan Scott defined second victims more broadly as "healthcare providers who are involved in an unanticipated adverse patient event, in a medical error and/or a patient related injury and become victimized in the sense that the provider is traumatized by the event" [45].

The National Quality Forum estimates that 1 million healthcare workers, including clinical, support, and administrative staff, have been directly or indirectly involved in events that led to patient harm [34]. However, it remains unclear how many experience second victim distress as a result. In one large study, 30% of physicians, nurses, and medical students surveyed reported mood symptoms or concerns about their ability to perform their jobs after a patient safety event [46]. In another study of pharmacists, nurses, and physicians, 43.4% reported anywhere from moderate to severe distress after making a medication error [64]. A more recent study showed that 57.9% of respondents, including physicians, nurses, pharmacists, social workers, and clinical technicians, reported second victim responses after an adverse patient incident [14].

Following adverse patient events, second victims may feel shame, guilt, anger, or loss of confidence [43, 62]. Clinicians may also experience psychiatric symptoms such as depressed mood, anxiety, or even suicidal ideation [5, 6, 28]. Symptoms such as sleep disturbances, difficulty concentrating, and lack of engagement can erode the well-being of providers, leading to even more errors [2, 48, 69]. The chance for committing medical errors has been reported to be elevated after clinicians experience the distress of the second victim experience [16, 50].

Second victims report that the impact of their distress can last months to years, with some never achieving full recovery [45, 54]. Some experience PTSD symptoms such as nightmares, flashbacks of the incident, and avoidance of situations associated with the error, leading to impairment in work performance and overall functioning [40, 70, 71]. Others may experience chronic fears of litigation or institutional punishment, decreased engagement with their work, a decline in job satisfaction, ultimately leading to burnout and thoughts of leaving the healthcare profession altogether [2, 16, 60]. One study showed a significant association between second victim distress and negative worker outcomes such as absenteeism or employees' plans to change jobs, particularly when organizational support was perceived to be low [2]. Frequent employee turnover and absenteeism are extremely costly to healthcare organizations. According to a study done in 2004, the average cost of losing and replacing a physician was estimated to be $123,000 in recruiting fees ($167,478 in 2020 currency) and $2 million in lost revenues ($2.7 million in 2020 currency) [32]. The cost of replacing a medical/surgical or specialty nurse was estimated to be $47,403 ($64,544 in 2020) and $85,197 ($116,005 in 2020), respectively [32]. As physician shortages increase in some specialties and chronic nursing shortages persist, strategies to minimize turnover may become even more critical [61].

Institutional Support for Second Victims

Increasingly aware of the high cost of the second victim phenomenon to providers, patient safety, and healthcare systems, several national organizations have called for institutional support of second victims. In 2010, the Joint Commission and the National Quality Forum recommended that health care institutions establish support structures to help healthcare works recover after traumatic events in the workplace [24, 34]. In a new policy outlined in July 2019, the American Medical Association encouraged physician wellness groups to consider developing peer support programs that are "voluntary, confidential, and non-discoverable." The new policy also encouraged further study of the prevalence and potential impact of the "second victim phenomenon" [78].

Despite these recommendations, there is evidence that effective institutional support remains limited. There have been numerous reports of clinicians who were highly distressed after medical errors and desired support but were unable to obtain it from their employers [5, 20, 22, 43, 58–60, 63]. In a survey study of 3171 physicians, 80% expressed interest in emotional support after a serious medical error, but only 10% felt adequately supported by their healthcare institutions [58].

This perceived lack of support is in notable contrast to what risk managers report about the availability of institutional support programs. In a survey of 575 risk managers in the United States, 73.6% reported that their hospitals had programs to provide emotional support to healthcare workers after adverse events [61]. However, 90.1% of these programs were housed within employee assistance programs (EAPs), and there are multiple reports in the literature indicating that clinicians, physicians in particular, infrequently turn to EAPs after adverse events [22, 29, 49]. Physicians have reported that barriers to seeking support from EAPs include fears of stigmatization given the perceived role of EAPs in addressing disruptive behavior, substance use, and performance issues [29]. This reluctance to seek help from EAPs may account for the divide between what providers and risk managers report about perceived institutional support.

Peer Support

Peer support has emerged in the literature as the preferred form of emotional support by second victims, rather than EAP services. Many institutions have found that healthcare workers across all disciplines desire peer support in the form of supportive and confidential discussion with colleagues when adverse patient events occur [22, 37, 46, 56]. It appears that distressed clinicians seek colleagues who will provide reassurance, compassion, active listening, and validation of their emotional responses [11]. Second victims also express benefit when a colleague can share similar experiences or put a medical error into perspective by framing it as a part of the profession or integral to the learning process [11, 36]. Commonly desired features of organizational support include prompt, easy access and a nonjudgmental, blame-free approach [11, 46].

Several healthcare institutions have established formal peer-support programs to address the needs of second victims. The peer support programs initiated by Brigham and Women's Hospital in 2004, University of Missouri in 2009, and Johns Hopkins University in 2011 have been early models for subsequent peer support programs in other hospital systems [11, 14, 27, 29, 30, 46, 49]. All three institutions have published papers about the design, implementation, and initial results of their programs [11, 14, 46, 49]. Table 8.1 is a comparative summary of the three programs. At all three institutions, multidisciplinary leadership teams conducted employee surveys to characterize the prevalence and needs of second victims, nominated and trained peer supporters, engineered peer support access based on the perceived needs of employees, and attempted to collect data regarding the peer support that was provided. However, there are notable differences between the programs that illustrate some of the challenges to providing effective organizational support to second victims.

Center for Professionalism and Peer Support at Brigham and Women's Hospital

Brigham and Women's Hospital's Center for Professionalism and Peer Support (CPPS) is one of the earliest peer support programs described in the literature. Established in 2004, CPPS initially provided multidisciplinary group peer support to distressed clinicians in which peer supporters had been trained by first responders such as emergency medical technicians. However, CPPS

Table 8.1 Summary of CPPS, RISE, and forYOU Peer Support Programs

	Brigham and Women's Hospital	Johns Hopkins Hospital	University of Missouri Health Care
Date founded	2004	2011 in pediatrics department 2012 hospital-wide	2009
Name of Program	Center for Professionalism and Peer Support (CPPS)	Resilience in Stressful Events (RISE)	forYOU
Leadership Team	- Physician director, physician associate director, and program manager	- Director of patient safety, a physician faculty member, a risk manager, a patient safety researcher, a nurse manager, and a hospital chaplain	- Representatives from patient safety, risk management, medical staff, nursing staff/managers, clergy, social sciences, respiratory therapy, the Employee Assistance Program, and education
Program Development	- Initially developed by Rick van Pelt, MD and Jane Barnes, RN, JD and provided group support to second victims	- Survey of frontline staff in pediatrics department (n = 144) - 70.8% nurses - 70% had been directly involved in adverse patient event - 57.9% reported mood problems or inability to perform job because of adverse patient event - 68.7% preferred multidisciplinary peers for support to other types of institutional support - 70.7% preferred individual to group support	- Studied other hospital programs including Brigham and Women's Hospital (CPPS) and Medically Induced Trauma Support Services in Boston, as well as nonhealthcare industry models such as Critical Incident Stress Management (CISM) used by aviation and first-responders after traumatic community events

- Survey demonstrated that physicians preferred support from physician colleagues rather than from multidisciplinary team because they had difficulty appearing vulnerable in front of nonphysicians - Decision was made in 2009 to redesign program to provide one-on-one support to second victims from professionally similar peers; group support still available	- Most commonly reported desired features of peer support program were: - Anonymity - Nonjudgmental approach - 24/7 access - Commitment to follow-up	- Qualitative study in which 31 healthcare providers who had been involved in event investigations were interviewed - Goal was to clarify and understand second victim experience - Gave rise to six stages of recovery for second victim, which shaped program design - Helped develop approach to screening second victims - Hospital-wide survey ($N = 898$) - 30% reported mood symptoms or concerns about ability to perform job after patient safety event - 15% seriously considered leaving profession after adverse patient event - 65% reported working out issue on their own; of those who reached out for support, 35% sought support from peers - Most frequently cited feature of support program was permission from institution to take time away from clinical area to regroup after adverse patient event - Next frequently cited was desire or just culture with "no-blame" mentality

(continued)

Table 8.1 (continued)

	Brigham and Women's Hospital	Johns Hopkins Hospital	University of Missouri Health Care

Program Design	- One-on-one or group peer support for any clinician or staff member involved in adverse patient event
	- First year of clinician self-referral yielded no calls
	- Switched to referral system: Clinicians referred confidentially by risk management, patient safety, and clinical leadership in event of known adverse events
	- Referral email sent to clinician, who can either accept or decline peer support
		- Timely one-on-one or group peer support offered to all employees after a stressful patient-related event
		- Clinician anonymously pages RISE team and receives response within 30 minutes, and is scheduled for an encounter within the next 12 hours
		- Two peer supporters available 24/7
		- RISE director available to provide additional support if technical or administrative issues arise
			- On-demand emotional support rapid response system that utilizes peer supporters and professional counseling for staff after adverse patient events
			- Three-tiered system to triage appropriate level of support
			- *Tier 1*: First responders
			  - Unit leaders and peers within departments trained to provide first-line surveillance and initial support for potential second victims and to identify emotionally challenging case types that are high risk for second victim response
			  - ForYOU team members available to provide real-time guidance for unit/department leaders if additional guidance is needed when supporting a colleague.
			- *Tier 2*: Support for second victims identified in Tier 1
			  - Individual or group emotional support provided by specially trained peer supporters
			  - Peers embedded in clinically high-risk departments such as OR, ICU, pediatrics, ED, trauma bay

			- *Tier 3*: Prompt escalation to professional counseling when peer support is inadequate - Professionals include chaplains, EAP personnel, social workers, and clinical psychologists - "Fast-track" referral within the institution provided - Tier 3 personnel mentor Tier 2 team members - Team leader on call 24/7 to support/coordinate peer supporters

Peer Supporter Training	- One half-day training focused on reflective listening, encouraging use of existing coping strategies, and providing additional resources	- Initial 6-hour training in psychological first aid
		- Monthly meetings in which peer supporters studied second victim literature, shared second victim encounters, and role-played support encounters
		- Debriefing after every peer encounter for additional support and supervision
			- 18 hours of didactics, small-group work, and simulation, covering the following topics:
			  - Second victim literature
			  - Institutional survey findings
			  - High-risk clinical events
			  - Six stages of second victim recovery
			  - Three-tiered system
			  - Active listening
			  - Referral procedures
			  - Monthly meetings for case reflection and mentoring

(continued)

Table 8.1 (continued)

	Brigham and Women's Hospital	Johns Hopkins Hospital	University of Missouri Health Care
Executive Support	- CPPS director reports directly to the Brigham and Women's Hospital's chief medical officer, who has supported the program since its inception by providing funding for leadership positions and ongoing financial support	- RISE leadership noted the program has relied on existing resources and has been reliant on voluntary efforts of staff, with limited funding for formal study of program outcomes	- Leaders from Missouri University Healthcare and from the University of Missouri School of Medicine have both supported and directly participated in the forYOU program, although their financial commitment is unclear
Clinician Engagement	- Brigham and Women's Hospital has about 8376 employees - Over a 4-year period, 240 clinicians received group peer support; 220 individual outreach calls made, but no data on how many of these individuals chose to receive peer support.	- Johns Hopkins Hospital has about 10,036 employees - Staff members who called RISE were not directly surveyed to preserve confidentiality and out of consideration of vulnerable emotional state; data collected below was from peer supporters who provided support	- University of Missouri Healthcare has about 6500 employees - To collect data below, peer supporters completed survey forms, NOT clinicians who sought support - 1075 total interventions documented over a 5-year period - 90.3% of clinicians' needs were addressed by Tier 1 or Tier 2 interventions - 9.7% of clinicians required Tier 3 professional counseling referrals

- Total number of clinicians supported by program unknown	- 119 calls over a 4.25-year period studied with data available for 80 of these calls:
	  - Nurse 56%
	  - Nurse practitioner 2.5%
	  - Multidisciplinary group 28.8%
	  - Physician 16.2%
	  - Other 6.3%
	  - Not recorded 13%
	- 4 of 80 incidents were related to a clear-cut medical error
		- 632 group support encounters
		  - 65% after unforeseen patient outcomes
		  - 33% related to personal or professional crisis
		  - 2% after adverse event related to medical error
		- 396 individual support encounters support
		  - 55% after unforeseen patient outcomes
		  - 28% related to personal or professional crisis
		  - 17% after adverse event related to medical error
		  - 53% Nurses or licensed practical nurses
		  - 23% Physicians, including attending, fellow, and resident physicians
		  - 17% allied health professionals, unlicensed staff members
		- 47 mentorship encounters between Tier 1 unit/department leaders and forYOU team

leadership noted that there was great reluctance by physicians to access the program because it appeared to be extremely challenging for physicians to acknowledge vulnerability before a multidisciplinary group that included nonphysicians [49]. In 2012, CPPS leaders conducted a survey study in which 88% of physicians stated that they preferred to receive support from other physician colleagues when needed [22]. This is consistent with data from two other studies in which the majority of physicians preferred to speak with other physicians after an error [36, 59]. In response, CPPS redesigned their peer support program to provide one-on-one peer support in which providers seeking help could be custom-matched with a peer clinician to accommodate physician preference for other physicians [49].

CPPS leaders nominated and trained clinical staff to be peer supporters, publicized the program within the hospital, and then invited distressed clinicians and staff to reach out to the program when needed. However, no clinicians requested support during the first year of the redesigned program [49]. A survey of their own physicians suggests possible reasons for the lack of clinician response. Nearly all of the physicians surveyed (89%) cited lack of time as a barrier to seeking needed emotional support. The majority also cited concerns about lack of confidentiality, negative impact on career, and the stigma of needing to access mental healthcare as barriers to seeking support [22]. In response to this data, CPPS leaders took a more pro-active approach to reaching distressed clinicians. Rather than waiting for employees to contact CPPS, staff from risk management, patient safety, and the employment assistance program made referrals directly to CPPS in the event of a known adverse event. CPPS then reached out to the provider [49].

While this is a commendably pro-active approach to reaching clinicians in need, distressed clinicians may perceive the referral as intrusive. Furthermore, given that the same department that conducts safety investigations is also making the referral for emotional support, it might be difficult for clinicians to fully disclose their responses to an event in an honest way. Providers referred in this way may not have enough institutional trust to fully engage with a peer support program in a way that is beneficial.

CPPS leaders reported that over a 3-year period, the program provided group peer support to 240 clinicians. In addition, 220 outreach calls to individual clinicians were made [49]. However, it is not stated how many of those referred to the program actually engaged in peer support services once offered. As such, it is impossible to fully assess how engaged employees were with the program. CPPS leaders expressed concern that that their program may not reach many clinicians who might benefit from it. They also acknowledged the need for outcome studies and have been developing a survey study to determine the effects of the program on second victims in their hospital system [49].

Resilience in Stressful Events (RISE) at Johns Hopkins Hospital

A multidisciplinary team at Johns Hopkins Hospital created the Resilience in Stressful Events (RISE) Program after patient safety leaders, risk management, and clinical departments began to recognize both the importance and the absence of consistent and timely support for second victims at their institution [15]. To address the needs of second victims, RISE leaders assembled a multidisciplinary team that included the hospital's patient safety director, a physician faculty member who has contributed significantly to the second victim literature, a risk manager, a patient safety researcher, a nurse manager, and a hospital chaplain [14]. A pre-implementation survey given to frontline staff in the pediatrics department in 2010 revealed that 66.4% had been directly involved in an adverse patient event, and 57.9% had experienced mood symptoms or difficulty performing their jobs after the event [14]. 70.7% of those surveyed preferred individual rather than group support, and 68.7% preferred support from peers rather than from nurse managers, pastoral care, counselors, or social workers [14]. RISE program leaders nominated and trained peer supporters, most of whom were nurses, but also included physicians, social workers, allied healthcare providers, patient safety staff, and a chaplain. RISE peer supporters had a higher level of support and supervision than was provided by the CPPS team for peer supporters at Brigham and Women's Hospital. In addition to an initial 6-hour training in psychological first aid, RISE peer supporters attended monthly meetings and debriefings after every peer encounter [14]. In contrast to the referral system used by CPPS, distressed clinicians at Johns Hopkins could anonymously page the RISE team anytime, 24 hours a day, 7 days a week, for a guaranteed response within 30 minutes to schedule an encounter within the next 12 hours [14]. This access system reflected the preferences of employees in the preimplementation survey, in which the most commonly desired features of a support program included anonymity and "24/7" access [11].

Similar to CPPS, RISE also received very few requests during the first year (12 calls). To increase clinician engagement, RISE leaders actively promoted the program in the hospital system through a dedicated website, publicity through internal publications, continuously cycling screen savers with program information, presentations to targeted departments and units, and recruitment of unit-level champions [14]. The volume of calls did increase over time, and by the time the program had been in place for 4.25 years, there had been 119 calls [14]. Similar to what happened at Brigham and Women's hospital, fewer physicians accessed the RISE program relative to other types of clinicians. Of the 80 calls with available data, 56% were made by nurses, while only 16.2% were made by physicians. The level of awareness of RISE was also significantly lower among physicians compared with nurses [11].

Four years after RISE had been established, program leaders conducted a post-implementation survey study in the pediatrics department. Mindful of confidentiality and the vulnerable emotional state of employees who activated peer support from RISE, the survey was distributed to all employees in the pediatrics department, not just to those who had sought peer support. This study showed that while more people were aware of RISE than when the pre-implementation survey was conducted, the percentage of people willing to access RISE was similar at both time points [11]. This suggests that despite the program's robust efforts to promote the program, some of the barriers cited by employees in the same study remained a challenge. Similar to the physicians at Brigham and Women's Hospital, employees in the pediatrics department at Johns Hopkins cited lack of time and the stigma of seeking emotional support as barriers to engage with RISE [11]. Others cited the need to overcome the culture of blame that persists in the hospital. One person in the study commented, "Getting people to use available resources when they have been used to just sucking it up is difficult. We need a culture change." Another stated, "I think there is still a stigma with using any resources like RISE…Despite what politically correct 'support' manager and others in the leadership may say, when it comes down to it, people tend to blame the victim rather than support [her/him]…" [11].

Blame vs. Just Hospital Cultures

Unfortunately, there is evidence that a blame culture is prevalent in many U.S. hospitals [17, 26]. A blame culture is characterized by employee unwillingness to accept responsibility for mistakes or take risks because of fear of criticism or management admonishment. Such a culture cultivates distrust and fear among providers, who then blame one other to avoid being reprimanded or belittled. As a result, clinician innovation and personal initiative suffer because the risk of being wrong among colleagues is perceived to be too high [26]. In this setting, silence is often the prevailing response to near misses or errors, especially when a provider from a high-status professional group commits the error [10, 35, 39, 52]. One can imagine that, by extension, distressed clinicians in a blame culture would be extremely hesitant to seek emotional support after an error. In a just culture, by contrast, organizations recognize the significant role that faulty systems play in medical errors, and they prioritize organizational learning over punitive treatment of individuals involved in errors [26]. The clinical milieu supports open dialogue regarding errors in order to promote safer practices [26]. Psychological safety is a critical element of a just culture, where providers feel they can question existing practices and admit mistakes without risking ridicule or punishment [53]. Amy Edmonson, who has written extensively about organizational learning and dynamics, particularly in complex, knowledge-driven industries such as healthcare, defines psychological safety as "a climate in which people are comfortable expressing and being themselves." In a psychologically safe environment, employees feel safe to share concerns or mistakes without the interpersonal risk of feeling humiliated, ignored, or blamed [12].

A large Belgian study demonstrated the significant impact that hospital culture can have on second victims. Van Gerven et al. found that a blame culture significantly increased the negative psychological impact on providers after a patient safety incident, whereas a supportive culture significantly reduced the psychological impact. Interestingly, the presence of second victim support programs did *not* influence psychological impact or recovery in this study, suggesting that hospital culture may have a more powerful impact on second victims than support programs [55].

The prevailing blame culture has also been strongly implicated as a major factor in the unacceptably high medical error rate in the United States, and some have argued that profound cultural change is a fundamental perquisite to making significant improvements in patient safety [7]. Hospital safety experts warn against a piecemeal approach to making patient safety changes, as these have shown a limited ability to promote a just culture throughout a healthcare system [38, 73, 74]. Rather, comprehensive changes that address culture and leadership, as well as specific components of care delivery, would be necessary [19]. It may be that to address hospital culture is also a fundamental prerequisite for an effective clinician support program for second victims. The limited engagement of clinicians in the CPPS and RISE programs may suggest that to have an organizational support program with robust clinician engagement, it must comprehensively shift culture and leadership, as well as local clinical practices.

The forYOU Rapid Response System for Second Victims at University of Missouri

In 2009, a team at University of Missouri Health Care (MUHC), led by Susan Scott, did just this by creating a comprehensive interventional support network for second victims, rather than a stand-alone peer support program. The program was named forYOU, and through its innovative 3-tiered design addressed many of the barriers to seeking care cited by healthcare workers such as lack of time and the stigma around seeking help [11, 22]. Not surprisingly, the forYOU program had markedly higher clinician engagement compared with the other peer support programs described in this chapter [11, 14, 46, 49].

The unique forYOU program design grew out of the 3-year period dedicated to understanding the second victim phenomenon and how it was affecting the staff at MUHC [46]. The forYOU team's extensive research and development period stands out among institutional peer support groups described in the literature in its thoroughness and clear commitment to try to understand the struggles and needs of second victims in their institution through both qualitative and quantitative studies. Similar to the RISE leadership team, the forYOU team was multidisciplinary and represented patient safety and risk management departments, medical and nursing staff, and clergy. In addition, the forYOU team included representatives from social work, respiratory therapy, education, and their EAP. After conducting an extensive literature review of the second victim experience, this interprofessional team then studied Brigham and Women's CPPS program, as well as Medically Induced Trauma Support Services (MITSS), a Massachusetts-based program that has provided a support network for patients, families, and clinicians following adverse medical events since 2002 [21, 46]. The forYOU team also explored support programs in non-healthcare industries for further guidance such as Critical Incident Stress Management (CISM), a program used in aviation and by pre-hospital first-responders after traumatic community events [21, 46]. The forYOU team incorporated Jean Watson's Theory of Transpersonal Care into their practice model. This is a holistic approach that encourages compassion, authentic presence, self-care, and an openness to spiritual and intuitive experiences when caring for patients [75].

After exploring various support models, the forYOU team conducted a year-long qualitative study in which they interviewed 31 healthcare providers (physicians, nurses, and allied healthcare professionals) who had been involved in patient safety event investigations. The goal of the study was to understand the second victim experience and to elicit specific healing interventions that participants believed would be most helpful in their recovery [44, 45]. An analysis of the qualitative data revealed that while participants had developed unique coping strategies, they also described recovery trajectories with similar features regardless of gender or professional group [44, 45]. Researchers delineated six stages of a predictable recovery pattern for second victims, which are summarized in Table 8.2. Stage 1, "chaos and response," begins as soon as an adverse event is identified. Clinicians experience chaos, confusion, and often a variety of stress-related physical and psychosocial symptoms. In Stage 2, "intrusive reflections," the second victim repeatedly replays and reflects upon the clinical event, often leading to feelings of inadequacy and isolation. Second victims in stage 3, "restoring personal integrity," experience intense fear about the impact of the error on his/her professional trajectory and on how he/she is perceived by colleagues. This leads to a search for acceptance and the need to regain trust from colleagues. Many clinicians find stage 4, "enduring the inquisition," to be extremely stressful, as this is the stage in which the second victim must recount the event during the investigation process. Fear and anxiety intensify as apprehension about future employment, career, and sometimes litigation grows. In Stage 5, "obtaining emotional first aid," second victims seek emotional support but experience uncertainty about how to find effective support and whom they can trust to discuss the event [44, 45].

Stage 6, "moving on," describes the ultimate outcome of the second victim's recovery path and can go in one of three possible directions: "dropping out," "surviving," or "thriving" [44, 45]. In dropping out, the second victim chooses to leave the practice environment by changing positions or even by leaving the healthcare profession altogether. Alternatively, the second victim may "survive" by continuing to work but also continuing to suffer from the event, never returning to pre-event baseline performance levels. The ideal outcome is of course thriving, in which second victims feel that they have gained valuable and transformative insights related to patient safety from the event. Many second victims who arrive at this stage actively participate in safety improvement plans to prevent future errors [44, 45].

Table 8.2 Second victim recovery stages

	Impact realization (individual may experience one or more of these stages simultaneously)					Moving on (individual migrates toward one of the three paths)		
Stage	Chaos and accident response	Intrusive reflections	Restoring personal integrity	Enduring the inquisition	Obtaining emotional first aid	Dropping out	Surviving	Thriving
Stage descriptors	- Point of impact is equal to event - Error recognized/error realized - Stabilize offering immediate supportive core for patient - May or may not be able to continue providing core for this patient - Clinician commonly distracted	- Evaluate clinical events that have transpired - Self-isolation to reflect on the case and care delivered - Haunted reenactments of event - Feelings of self-doubt and professional inadequacies - Shock and denial	- Fears rejection among work/social structure - Fear of the unknown (next steps) is prevalent - Struggling to get back to "baseline" level of professional skill confidence	- Realization of event severity - Reiterate scenario - Respond to numerous clinical questions surrounding the event - Interact with event responders (many strangers)	- Identify who is safe to confide in - Attempting personal/professional support - May 'hint and hope' for support from various sources	- Feelings of inadequacy and failure - Leave current role by transferring to different facility or unit - Consider quitting profession altogether	- Coping with what has transpired - Persistent sadness prevails - Trying to learn from event - Assist in defense of legal action	- Does not base practice/work on one event - Minimal adverse effect from event - Advocates for patient safety initiatives - Tries to make a difference for the next patient or clinician

(continued)

Table 8.2 (continued)

	Impact realization (individual may experience one or more of these stages simultaneously)					Moving on (individual migrates toward one of the three paths)		
Stage	Chaos and accident response	Intrusive reflections	Restoring personal integrity	Enduring the inquisition	Obtaining emotional first aid	Dropping out	Surviving	Thriving
Second victim's personal goals	- Recognize event occurred	- Conceptualize and understand what has transpired	- Restore personal/professional credibility among peers and supervisors	- Provide effective accounts of the event	- Identify a safe zone to communicate feelings regarding the event	- Determine future professional role	- Identify ways to cope from impact of the event	- Identify ways to process the event and make a positive impact on future events
Institutional supportive objectives	- Identify potential second victims Assess staff (s)' ability to continue shift - Determine if second victim support is needed	- Identify key individuals involved in the event - Formalize a second victim response plan - Observe staff for lingering physical or psychological symptoms	- Provide oversight of event and manage overall response including gossip control - Evaluate if a team debrief would be beneficial	- Start to collect all details of what happened from key event participants - Develop understanding of what happened and begin formulating "why" did it happen and could it be prevented - Document event investigation according to institution policies	- Ensure that optimal emotional support is offered - Assure risk management and patient safety resources are available as needed	- Provide ongoing support of the second victim and maintain dialogue - If needed, assist the second victim in search for alternative employment options	- Provide ongoing support of the second victim and maintain dialogue	- Provide ongoing support of the second victim - Support second victim in how to make a difference for future events including mentoring others in similar situations

Risk management interventions	- Gather information and start preclaim file	- Talk to staff involved and allow venting of concerns	- Contact with the staff discussing event and status of investigation - Encouraging staff not to allow event to change good practice techniques - Provide information to legal counsel and insurance	- Discuss case details with staff to preserve information for risk management/legal use - Assistance with disclosure, apology, offer of compensation to patient/family, work with billing issues as needed - Assurance to staff of support during all phases of investigation and anxiety	- Answer questions about investigations or litigation process, what to expect, and assistance available - Discuss personal and family counseling options inside and outside the organization	- Provide medical malpractice information as needed by staff for licensure, credentialing, and other applications	- Supporting and working with staff on the defense of the legal action - Working with internal and/or external attorneys	- Identify staff who have survived an event to mentor a peer who might be going through a similar experience

Adapted with permission from [44]

ForYOU leaders used this nuanced understanding of the second victim recovery stages to guide their design of interventions for their peer support program. Similar to the CPPS and RISE programs, they also conducted a survey of their employees to characterize the second victim experience and to find out what features employee were looking for in a support program. Of the 898 respondents, 30% reported mood symptoms or concerns about their ability to perform their jobs as a result of a clinical patient safety event, and 15% of this group had seriously contemplated leaving their chosen professions [46]. Reflecting concerns that clinicians tend to suffer in silence, 65% of employees who reported suffering after adverse patient events reported that they did not seek out support [46]. The survey also included opportunities for narrative response about what employees believed would be helpful from an organizational support program and identified eight common themes that described characteristics of an ideal program [46]. Employees most frequently cited wanting to have an institutionally sanctioned respite away from the clinical environment immediately after an event so that a second victim could try to regain composure in private. The next most commonly cited feature was a safe and just culture approach with a no-blame mentality [46]. Based on this large survey, forYOU team leaders concluded that MUHC healthcare workers wanted formal organizational support, ideally at the departmental or unit level, that includes prompt, confidential, and easy access to professionally trained counselors [46].

The Scott Three-Tiered Integrated Model

Once the forYOU team presented the extensive data collected from their literature review, their study of multiple support models, and their interview and survey results, MUHC senior leaders overwhelmingly supported the establishment of a formal program to provide emotional support to second victims. The forYOU team then developed the Scott Three-Tiered Integrated Model to provide rapid, on-demand emotional support to second victims 24 hours a day, 7 days a week [46]. In contrast to the stand-alone peer support programs described by other institutions in the literature, the forYOU program is a flexible and comprehensive second victim support network that provides varying levels of support to distressed clinicians. The overall structure of the Scott Three-Tiered Integrated Model of Second Victim Support is illustrated in Fig. 8.1.

Tier 1 was designed to provide surveillance and initial support for potential second victims at the unit or departmental level. Based on the six stages of second victim recovery that emerged from their interview data, the forYOU team trained individual unit leaders and select peers from within departments to identify both second victims and emotionally challenging case types that put clinicians at high risk for experiencing second victim symptoms [21, 46]. The forYOU team trained department leaders and peers working on the unit to administer immediate psychological first aid for distressed clinicians once identified [21, 46]. ForYOU team members are also available to provide real-time assistance for unit/department leaders if additional guidance is needed when supporting a colleague [21].

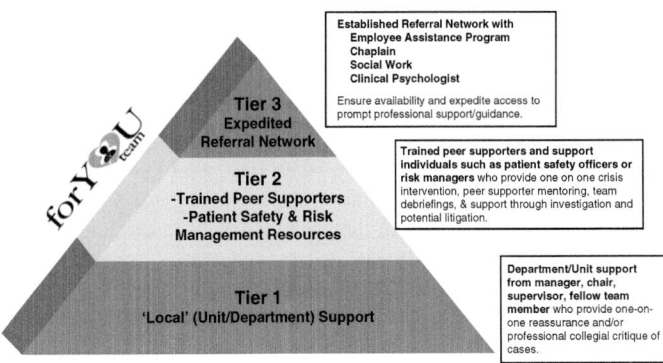

Fig. 8.1 The Scott Three-Tiered Interventional Model of Second Victim Support. (Reproduced with permission from [46])

The active involvement of leaders as trained peers at the unit level is perhaps one of the most powerful and innovative features of the Scott 3-Tier Method. Training unit and department leaders to identify second victims and intervene quickly with sensitive emotional support normalizes clinician distress after adverse events and very likely reduces the stigma around seeking support, a commonly cited barrier for engaging in peers support programs [11, 21, 22, 49]. Moreover, unit leaders who survey their colleagues for distress and intervene with timely and sensitive emotional support, particularly when the adverse event involves medical error, potentially shift the culture at the local level from a blame culture to a just culture by increasing the psychological safety of the unit. By affecting both culture change and leadership, the forYOU program exemplifies the kind of comprehensive change that many patient safety experts recommend for an effective shift from a blame to a just culture [19, 23].

In Tier 2, individual or group emotional support is provided by trained peer supporters to second victims identified in Tier 1 [46]. Peer supporters include physicians, nurses, social workers, and allied health professionals, and their training is considerably more extensive than what has been described by other programs in the literature, including CPPS and RISE [11, 14, 21, 46, 49]. ForYOU peer supporter training includes 18 hours of didactics, small-group sessions, and simulations, as well as monthly meetings for case reflection and additional mentoring. Peer supporters learn critical incident stress management techniques and to identify high-risk clinical events that are more likely to elicit a second victim response [21, 46]. Initially, forYOU peer supporters were recruited from and placed in departments that are clinically high risk for second victim reactions, such as operating rooms, intensive care units, pediatrics departments, and the emergency department/trauma bay. This is a particularly strategic approach, as it facilitates recognition of second victims in areas of the hospital that are most likely to have the largest numbers of second victims. Having trusted colleagues who are sensitive to clinician distress further normalizes the second victim experience. Clinicians might be more accepting of help and feel less stigmatized when everyone on the unit is offered support after an adverse event, not just individuals involved in safety investigations. Having peer supporters embedded on units also removes the burden of navigating an access system for distressed clinicians seeking peer support, which was cited as a barrier to seeking help by second victims in previous studies [11, 22]. Many providers have also cited lack of time as a significant barrier to seeking needed support [11, 22, 46]. The forYOU program addresses this by providing immediate, on-site support when needed, without the need to schedule a peer support session outside of work hours.

Tier 2 peer supporters can also refer second victims to other resources available within the hospital. They can refer colleagues to patient safety experts for support during the immediate aftermath of a patient safety event and any institutional investigation that may follow, or to risk management for guidance in the event of litigation [46]. Peer supporters may also escalate care to Tier 3 if they feel that a distressed colleague requires a higher level of emotional support than they feel equipped to provide. Tier 3 is a "fast-track" referral source to professional counselors within the institution. Tier 3 professionals include chaplains, EAP personnel, social workers, and clinical health psychologists [46]. These providers also serve as mentors to Tier 2 peer support rapid response team members [21]. This creates a symbiotic relationship in which Tier 2 peer supporters gain additional supervision from experienced clinicians while Tier 3 providers gain increased experience and understanding of the profound emotional trauma that many experience after an adverse patient event [46]. Given the aforementioned preference that many physicians have for receiving support from other physicians, clinician engagement may improve if psychiatrists are among the Tier 3 providers [22, 49].

Five years after implementing their program, the forYOU team created a data collection tool and distributed it to forYOU peer supporters after activations and during monthly team meetings to evaluate the program's effectiveness [21]. Presumably out of the same concern the RISE program had for maintaining confidentiality and emotional sensitivity for those who had sought support, the forYOU leaders did not directly survey second victims who received support. Informal Tier 1 interactions were not monitored or included in this survey. The survey results indicated that Tier 2 interventions addressed the needs of 90.3% of MUHC clinicians who had received peer support, and 9.7% required Tier 3 professional referrals [21]. Overall provider engagement with forYOU was markedly greater than what was reported by CPPS or RISE. Over the course of 5 years, there were 1075 documented support encounters [21]. The forYOU program was available to 6500 employees in the University of Missouri Health Care system [21]. CPPS at Brigham and Women's Hospital reported that over a 3-year period, 240 clinicians received group peer support, while 220 outreach calls were made to clinicians who were involved in patient safety investigations [49]. However, because it is not known how many of these outreach calls resulted in individual peer support encounters, it is not known exactly how many clinicians utilized the program.

Nonetheless, considering that Brigham and Women's Hospital is a larger healthcare system, with around 8500 employees, this was still a lower level of clinician engagement relative to the forYOU program [1]. The RISE program had even less robust clinician engagement. After 4.25 years, out of the approximately 10,000 employees at Johns Hopkins Hospital, 119 calls to RISE were reported [14, 77]. Team leaders from both RISE and CPPS cited getting staff members who need support to utilize their programs to be the greatest challenge to their programs [11, 14, 49].

There are certainly many possible reasons that clinician engagement was so much higher with the forYOU program compared with other programs. Recognizing that further studies would need to be done to demonstrate this, our hypothesis is that the forYOU program was more successful in engaging its employees because the design of the program actively promoted a just culture by training unit leaders to offer emotional first aid to suspected second victims and by embedding highly trained peer supporters in the clinical milieu. This shift toward increased psychological safety addresses a significant barrier to seeking help expressed by many second victims in multiple studies, namely the shame and stigma associated with both experiencing second victim symptoms after an adverse patient event and seeking help. Creating a culture of psychological safety has already been demonstrated to be a key component of making lasting and effective changes to patient safety [47, 57]. It may be that may be that a culture shift toward psychological safety is equally important in creating effective support systems for distressed caregivers. Given that distressed second victims are at higher risk for making errors, providing support to second victims is arguably also a patient safety initiative [2].

Although the forYOU program had overall greater clinician engagement, there were some trends in the way clinicians utilized support that were similar to what was reported by CPPS and RISE. Similar to CPPS and RISE, fewer physicians sought support from the forYOU program relative to other types of providers. Of the one-on-one Tier 2 interventions that were reported in the 5-year post-implementation survey, 53% were for nursing staff, 23% were for physicians (including attending, fellow, and resident physicians), and 17% were for allied health professionals and nonclinical staff [21]. Similar to what was reported by RISE, the smallest proportion of forYOU activations were for adverse events related to medical error. 17% of the Tier 2 encounters were for medical error, 28% for personal/professional crisis, and 55% for unforeseen/unanticipated patient outcomes [21]. These trends highlight the ongoing challenge of providing support to physicians and to all clinicians after a medical error. Qualitative studies may be helpful to try to characterize what type of interventions physicians would utilize, given the barriers to seeking care they have described, such as lack of time, concerns about confidentiality, and the stigma of needing to access mental healthcare. Some have argued that a deep-seated culture of shame that endures in medical training may create a particularly persistent barrier to physicians reaching out for support when needed, particularly in the case of medical error [41, 76]. Given the tendency of providers to isolate when feeling shame, they may continue to suffer in silence until shame in clinical and educational culture is addressed [41].

Future Directions

Team leaders from CPPS, RISE, and forYOU acknowledge the need for further studies to assess the long-term effectiveness of their programs and to delineate which features of programs second victims find most helpful [14, 46, 49]. It is possible that clinician engagement will improve over time, but over a longer interval than the 3–5 year periods measured in the current studies of these programs. It would be important to know if peer support programs reduce mood symptoms and burnout in providers, or if providing institutional support for second victims decreases the number of errors.

In addition, the challenges faced by the three support programs described here underscore both the importance and the difficulty of changing the culture of shame and blame in the clinical environment. Pre-implementation surveys of employees to characterize second victim distress should also include items that allow providers to describe their perceptions of the clinical culture in which they work. Burlison et al. have developed an assessment called the Second Victim Experience and Support Tool (SVEST) that includes questions about perceived colleague, supervisor, and institutional support that can be used to help gauge employees' perceptions of the psychological safety of the culture of an institution [3]. Tools such a as this could be used as a starting point in assessing whether a just vs. blame culture is present. A possible challenge with such surveys is clinician concern about lack of anonymity or reprisal for reporting a blame culture. The shift from blame to just culture is admittedly an even more complex process, with even fewer guidelines for best practices than are available for addressing second victim distress. However, creating a second victim support program without simultaneously addressing the culture of blame and shame that prevails in many institutions may result in limited clinician engagement, as the programs discussed in this chapter have found.

The issue of confidentiality in peer support programs is also a significant hurdle that must be cleared in order for clinicians to feel comfortable engaging in existing peer support programs.

Respondents to surveys conducted by CPPS, RISE, and forYOU programs all expressed the importance of confidentiality in seeking peer support, with many physicians in particular citing concerns about confidentiality as a major barrier to seeking support when needed [11, 14, 22, 46, 49]. In the CPPS and RISE programs, peer intervention confidentiality is broken only in the case in which there is a concern that the distressed victim may be an acute danger to self or other [14, 49]. It would be useful to clarify this with hospital staff when introducing any peer support program.

However, a murkier and more problematic element of confidentiality in peer interventions is discoverability in the case of future litigation for a medical error. Laws regarding protected status for peer support interactions are unclear and vary highly from state to state, and this ambiguity may deter second victims from seeking help, especially given the looming specter of malpractice that shapes communications following adverse events [72]. Ideally, unambiguous and comprehensive protections should be incorporated into existing federal legislation such as the Patient Safety and Quality Improvement Act [72]. Without some sort of clear legislation to protect communications for second victims support interventions, fears about confidentiality may remain a significant barrier to providers seeking emotional support after adverse patient events. This would be especially true for physicians, who tend to bear the brunt of legal responsibility following an adverse patient event that proceeds to litigation. While a psychologically unsafe work environment has been implicated in the culture of silence around healthcare providers reporting medical errors and seeking emotional support in the aftermath of such errors, provider fears about confidentiality in the case of litigation also likely contribute significantly to this silence [26, 72]. CPPS managed the legal ambiguity of confidentiality by not keeping written notes of peer support interventions [49]. However, not having any documentation of peer encounters impedes further training and supervision of peer supporters, as well as much-needed evaluation of support programs to assess and improve their effectiveness.

As the urgency for healthcare organizations to address both provider burnout and patient safety mounts, designing effective support programs for second victims can appear to be an insurmountable enterprise, given the challenges and complexities of doing so effectively as reflected by the experiences of the three programs discussed in this chapter. However, leaders from these programs have demonstrated the initiative, creativity, and persistence needed to approach this daunting and critical task. Team leaders from CPPS, RISE, and forYOU identified second victim syndrome as a problem and brought it to the attention of senior leadership at their institutions, and it is important to note that all three programs had strong support from hospital leadership [11, 14, 21, 44, 46, 49]. Committed executive leadership and the allocation of appropriate resources are critical to providing comprehensive second victim support [9, 34, 48]. Patient safety experts have stressed the importance of involving senior leadership in implementing any lasting changes to improve patient safety [19]. After securing executive buy-in, leaders of CPPS, RISE, and forYOU then conducted studies to better understand the prevalence and characteristics of second victims in their own institutions, as well as what features they preferred from a support system. This allowed each organization to engage in an iterative design and implementation process in which interventions were tailored to the specific needs of its employees. Program leaders noted the lack of existing literature about necessary steps to implement second victim support programs, as well as an absence of any outcome studies for existing programs [14, 46]. Rather than using the dearth of evidence about best practices as a reason to maintain the status quo as many institutions unfortunately do, these team leaders took daring steps to design their own programs, refine and study them, and then publish the process and results so that others can benefit from lessons learned. This thoughtful and imaginative approach should serve as a model to other institutions that have identified the need for organizational support programs for second victims but are waiting for evidence for best practices to appear in the literature to start their own support programs. Addressing second victim syndrome is a complex problem that will require resources, creativity, and the willingness to experiment with novel programs. Healthcare institutions can hardly afford to take a less proactive approach given the high cost of second victim distress to providers, patient safety, and a sustainable healthcare workforce.

References

1. Bloomberg. Brigham and Women's Hospital Inc. 2020. Accessed from https://www.bloomberg.com/profile/company/3667869Z:US on 30 Dec 2019.
2. Burlison JD, Quillivan RR, Scot SD, Johnson S, Hoffman JM. The effects of the second victim phenomenon on work-related outcomes: connecting self-reported caregiver distress to turnover intentions and absenteeism. J Patient Saf. 2016;1(10):1–13.
3. Burlison JD, Scott SD, Browne EK, Thompson SG, Hoffman JM. The second victim experience and support tool: validation of an organizational resource for assessing second victim effects and the quality of support resources. J Patient Saf. 2017;13(2):93–102.
4. Carr S. Disclosure and apology: what's missing? Advancing programs that support clinicians. Boston: Medically Induced Trauma Support services, Inc.; 2009.
5. Christensen JF, Levinson W, Dunn PM. The heart of darkness. J Gen Intern Med. 1992;7:424–31.
6. Pronovost PJ, Bienvenu OJ. From shame to guilt to love. JAMA. 2015;314:2507–8.
7. Cohen MM, Eustis MA, Gribbins RE. Changing the culture of patient safety: leadership's role in health care quality and improvement. Jt Comm J Qual Saf. 2003;29(7):329–35.
8. Conway J, Federico F, Stewart K, et al. Respectful management of serious clinical adverse events. Cambridge, MA: Institute for Healthcare Improvement; 2011.
9. Denham CR. TRUST: the 5 rights of the second victim. J Patient Saf. 2007;3(2):107–19.
10. Detert JR, Edmondson AC. Why employees are afraid to speak up. Harvard Business Review. 2007;23–25.
11. Dukhanin V, Edrees HH, Connors C, Kang E, Norvell M, Wu AW. Case: a second victim support program in pediatrics: successes and challenges to implementation. J Pediatr Nurs. 2018;41:54–9.
12. Edmondson AC. The fearless organization: creating psychological safety in the workplace for learning, innovation, and growth. Hoboken: Wiley; 2019.

13. Edrees HH, Morlock L, Wu AW. Do hospitals support second victims? Collective insights from patient safety leaders in Maryland. Jt Comm J Qual Patient Saf. 2017;43:471–83.
14. Edrees HH, Connors C, Paine L, Norvell M, Taylor H, Wu AW. Implementing the RISE second victim support programme at the Johns Hopkins Hospital: a case study. BMJ. 2016;6:e011708.
15. Edrees HH, Paine LA, Feroli ER, Wu AW. Health care workers as second victims of medical errors. Pol Arch Med Wewn. 2011;121:101–8.
16. Fahrenkopf AM, Sectish TC, Barger LK, Sharek PJ, Lewin D, Chiang VW, et al. Rates of medication errors among depressed and burnt out residents: prospective cohort study. Br Med J. 2008;336:488–91.
17. Farley DO, Haviland A, Champagne S, Jain AK, Battles JB, Munier WB, et al. Adverse-event reporting practices by US hospitals: results of a national survey. Qual Saf Health Care. 2009;17:416–23.
18. Firth S. AMA to promote use of peer support groups. 2019, June 13. Retrieved from https://www.medpagetoday.com/meetingcoverage/ama/80467 on 28 Dec 2019.
19. Frankel A, Gandhi TK, Bates DW. Improving patient safety across a large integrated health care delivery system. International J Qual Health Care. 2003;15(Suppl. 1):i31–40.
20. Gallagher TH, Waterman AD, Ebers AG. Patients' and physicians' attitudes regarding the disclosure of medical errors. JAMA. 2003;289:1001–7.
21. Hirschinger LR, Scott SD, Hahn-Cover K. Clinician support: five years of lessons learned. Patient Saf Qual Healthc. 2015;12(2):26–31.
22. Hu YY, Fix ML, Hevelone ND, et al. Physicians' needs in coping with emotional stressors: the case for peer support. Arch Surg. 2012;147:212–7.
23. Institute of Medicine. Keeping patients safe: transforming the work environment of nurses. Washington, DC: The National Academy Press; 2004.
24. Joint Commission. Looking at sentinel events along the continuum of patient safety. Joint Commission Perspectives. 2010;30(8). 3–5. from RISE nursing paper.
25. Johns Hopkins University Hospital, Department of Human Resources. Employee head count and full time equivalent as of 1/1/2018. 2018, January 1. Accessed from https://www.hopkinsmedicine.org/human_resources/about/employee_numbers.html on 30 Dec 2019.
26. Khatri N, Brown GD, Hicks LL. From a blame culture to a just culture in health care. Health Care Manage Rev. 2009;34(4):312–22.
27. Krzan KD, Merandi J, Morvay S, Mirtallo J. Implementation of a "second victim" program in a pediatric hospital. Am J Health Sys Pharm. 2015;72:563–7.
28. Lander LI, Connor JA, Shah RK, Kentala E, Healy GB, Roberson DW. Otolaryngologists' responses to errors and adverse events. Laryngoscope. 2006;116:1114–20.

29. Lane MA, Newman BM, Taylor MZ, O'Neill M, Getti C, Wotman RM, Waterman AD. Supporting clinicians after adverse events: development of a clinician peer support program. J Patient Saf. 2018;14(5):56–60.
30. Majed WE, Bohnen JD, Westfal M, Han K, Cauley C, Wright C, Schulz J, Mort E, Ferris T, Lillemoe KD, Kaafarani H. Design and impact of a novel surgery-specific second victim peer support program. J Am Coll Surg. 2020;230:926–33.
31. Merandi JM, Liao N, Lewe D, Morvay S, Stewart B, Catt C, Scott S. Deployment of a second victim peer support program: a replication study. Pediatr Qual Saf. 2017;2:1–8.
32. Misra-Hebert A, Kay R, Stoller J. A review of physician turnover: rates, causes, an consequences. Am J Med Qual. 2004;19(2):56–66.
33. Mitzman J, Jones C, Mcnamara S, et al. Curated collection for educators: five key papers about second victim syndrome. Cureus. 2019;11(3):e4186. https://doi.org/10.7759/cureus.4186.
34. National Quality Forum. Safe practices for better healthcare—2010 update: a consensus report. https://www.qualityforum.org/Publications/2010/04/Safe_Practices_for_Better_Healthcare_%E2%80%93_2010_Update.aspx. 2010. Accessed 2 Jan 2020.
35. Nembhard IM, Edmondson AC. Making it safe: the effects of leader inclusiveness and professional status on psychological safety and improvement efforts in healthcare teams. J Organ Behav. 2006;27:941–66.
36. Plews-Ogan M, May N, Owens J, Ardelt M, Shapiro J, Bell SK. Wisdom in medicine: what helps physicians after a medical error? Acad Med. 2016;91:233–41.
37. Pratt S, Kenney L, Scott SD, Wu AW. How to develop a second victim support program: a toolkit for health care organization. Joint Comm J Qual and Patient Saf. 2012;38(5):235–40.
38. Pronovost PJ, Weast B, Holzmueller CG, Rosenstein BJ, Kidwell RP, Haller KB, et al. Evaluation of the culture of safety: survey of clinicians and managers in an academic medical center. Qual Saf Health Care. 2003;12:405–10.
39. Ramanujam R, Rousseau DM. The challenges are organizational not just clinical. J Organ Behav. 2006;27:811–27.
40. Rassin M, Kanti T, Silner D. Chronology of medication errors by nurses: accumulation of stresses and PTSD symptoms. Issues Ment Health Nurs. 2005;26:873–86.
41. Robertson JJ, Brit L. Suffering in slience: medical errors and its impact on health care providers. J Emerg Med. 2018;54(4):402–9.

42. Schiff G, Griswold P, Ellis BR, et al. Doing right by our patients when things go wrong in the ambulatory setting. Jt Comm J Qual Patient Saf. 2014;40:91–6.
43. Schwappah DL, Boluarte TA. The emotional impact of medical error involvement on physicians: a call for leadership and organizational accountability. Swiss Med Wkly. 2009;139:9–15.
44. Scott SD, McCaoic MM. Care at the point of impact: insights into the second-victim experience. J Healthc Risk Manag. 2016;35(4):6–13.
45. Scott SD, Hirschinger LE, Cox KR, McCoig MM, Brandt J, Hall LW. The natural history of recovery for the healthcare provider second victim after adverse patient events. J Qual Saf Health Care. 2009;18:325–30.
46. Scott SD, Hirschinger LE, Cox K, McCoig M, Hahn-Cover K, Epperly KM, Phillips EC, Hall LW. Caring for our own: deploying a systemwide second victim rapid response team. Joint Comm J Qual and Patient Saf. 2010;35:233–40.
47. Scott-Cawiezell J, Jones K, Moore L, Vojir C. Nursing home culture: a critical component of sustained improvement. J Nurs Care Qual. 2004;20:341–8.
48. Seys D, Wu AW, VanGerven E, Vleugels A, Euwema M, Panella M, et al. Healthcare professionals as second victims after adverse events: a systematic review. Eval Health Prof. 2013;36(2):133–60.
49. Shapiro J, Galowtiz P. Peer support for clinicians: a programmatic approach. Acad Med. 2016;91:1200–4.
50. Shanafelt TD, Balch CM, Bechamps G, et al. Burnout and medical errors among American surgeons. Ann Surg. 2010;251(6):995–1000.
51. Tamburri LM. Creating healthy work environments for second victims of adverse events. AACN Crit Care. 2017;24(4):366–73.
52. Tangirala S, Ramanujam R. Employee silence on critical work issues: the cross level effects of procedural justice climate. Pers Psychol. 2008;61(1):37–68.
53. Tucker AL, Nembhard IM, Edmondson AC. Implementing new practices: an empirical study of organizational learning in hospital intensive care units. Manag Sci. 2007;53:894–907.
54. Ullström S, Andreen SM, Hansson J, Øvretveit J, Brommels M. Suffering in silence: a qualitative study of second victims of adverse events. BJM Qual Saf. 2014;23(4):325–31.
55. Van Gerven E, Bruyneel L, Panella M, Euwema M, Sermeus W, Vanhaecht K. Psychological impact and recovery after involvement in a patient safety incident: a repeated measures analysis. BMJ Open. 2016;6(8):e011403.
56. van Pelt F. Peer support: healthcare professionals supporting each other after adverse medical events. Qual Saf Health Care. 2008;17:249–52.
57. Vestal KW, Fralicx RD, Spreier SW. Organizational culture: the critical link between strategy and results. Hosp Health Serv Adm. 1997;42:339–65.

58. Waterman AD, Garbutt J, Hazel E, et al. The emotional impact of medical errors on practicing physicians in the United States and Canada. Jt Comm J Qual Patient Saf. 2007;33:467–76.
59. West CP, Huschka MM, Novotny PJ, et al. Association of perceived medical errors with resident distress and empathy: a prospective longitudinal study. JAMA. 2006;296:1071–8.
60. West CP, Tan AD, Habermann TM, Sloan JA, Shanafelt TD. Association of resident fatigue and distress with perceived medical errors. JAMA. 2009;302:1294–300.
61. White AA, Brock DM, McCotter PI, Hofeldt R, Edrees HH, Wu AW, Shannon S, Gallagher TH. Risk managers' descriptions of programs to support second victims after adverse events. J Healthc Risk Manag. 2015;34(4):30–40. https://doi.org/10.1002/jhrm.21169.
62. White AA, Gallagher TH. After the apology-coping and recovery after errors. Virtual Mentor. 2011;13(9):593–600.
63. White AA, Waterman A, McCotter P, Boyle D, Gallagher TH. Supporting health care workers after medical error: considerations for health care leaders. J Clin Outcomes Manag. 2008;15(5):240–7.
64. Wolf ZR, Serembus JF, Smetzer J, Cohen H, Cohen M. Response and concerns of healthcare providers to medication errors. Clin Nurse Spec. 2000;14:278–87.
65. Wu AW. Medical error: the second victim: the doctor who makes the mistake needs help too. BMJ. 2000;320(7237):726–7.
66. Wu AW, Folkman S, McPhee SJ, et al. Do house officers learn from their mistakes? JAMA. 1991;265:2089–94.
67. Wears RL, Wu AW. Dealing with failure: the aftermath of errors and adverse events. Ann Emerg Med. 2002;39(3):344–346. https://doi.org/10.1067/mem.2002.121996.
68. Shanafelt TD, Boone S, Tan L, et al. Burnout and satisfaction with work-life balance among US physicians relative to the general US population. Arch Intern Med. 2012;172(18):1377–1385. https://doi.org/10.1001/archinternmed.2012.3199.
69. Quillivan RR, Burlison JD, Browne EK, Scott SD, Hoffman JM. Patient Safety Culture and the Second Victim Phenomenon: Connecting Culture to Staff Distress in Nurses. Jt Comm J Qual Patient Saf. 2016;42(8):377–86. https://doi.org/10.1016/s1553-7250(16)42053-2. PMID:27456420; PMCID: PMC5333492.
70. Scott SD, Hirschinger LE, Cox KR. Sharing the load. Rescuing the healer after trauma. RN. 2008;71(12):38–43.
71. Schelbred AB, Nord R. Nurses' experiences of drug administration errors. J Adv Nurs. 2007;60(3):317–324. https://doi.org/10.1111/j.1365-2648.2007.04437.x.
72. de Wit ME, Marks CM, Natterman JP, Wu AW. Supporting second victims of patient safety events: shouldn't these communications be covered by

legal privilege?. J Law Med Ethics. 2013;41(4):. https://doi.org/10.1111/jlme.12095.
73. Cook AF, Hoas H, Guttmannova K, Joyner JC. An error by any other name. Am J Nurs. 2004;104(6):32–44. https://doi.org/10.1097/00000446-200406000-00025.
74. Institute of Medicine (US) Committee on Quality of Health Care in America. Crossing the Quality Chasm: A New Health System for the 21st Century. Washington (DC): National Academies Press (US); 2001.
75. Watson, J. Nursing-The philosophy and science of caring. Boulder: F.A. Davis Company; 2008.
76. Robertson JJ, Long B. Medicine's Shame Problem. J Emerg Med. 2019;57(3):329–338. https://doi.org/10.1016/j.jemermed.2019.06.034.
77. Employee Head Count and Full Time Equivalents as of 1/1/2020. Johns Hopkins Medicine website. January 1, 2020. Accessed January 15, 2020. https://www.hopkinsmedicine.org/human_resources/about/employee_numbers.html.
78. American Medical Association House of Delegates. 2019 Meeting: Memorial resolutions adopted unanimously. Updated November 17, 2019. Accessed December 30, 2019. https://www.ama-assn.org/system/files/2020-01/a19-resolutions.pdf.

Index

A
Access to Recovery (ATR), 22
Affordable Care Act, 50
Alcoholics Anonymous (AA), 7

B
Bandura's Social Learning Theory, 135
Bereaved individuals
  peer support
    careful selection, 84, 85
    confidentiality, 82
    definition, 73
    desirable qualities, 87–89
    easily accessible and responsive, 82
    grief symptoms, 75
    hopeful reappraisal phase, 78, 79
    internet based support, 89, 90
    monitoring and care, 86, 87
    organizational case study, 75
    person receiving support, 83, 84
    positive integration, 80–82
    professional mental health care providers, 85
    safe environment, 83
    social support, 73, 74
    stabilization phase, 76, 77
    TAPS, 75, 76
    training, 85, 86
  prevalence, 71
BlueStar™, 63

C
Center for Professionalism and Peer Support (CPPS), 156, 157
Certified Older Adult Peer Specialists (COAPS) program, 122
Chronic care model (CCM), 58–61
Chronic illness
  peer education, 97, 98
  peer influence, 96
  peer interventions, 97–99
  peer support
    appraisal support, 96
    development and implementation, 103
    emotional support, 96
    face-to-face peer support, 101
    formative evaluation, 104
    HRQoL, 101
    informational support, 96
    matching mentors and adolescents, 104

Chronic illness (*cont.*)
    mode of delivery, 104–106
    peer-led camp program, 102
    peer mentors/educators, 106–108
    positive role models, 100
    problem-solving training, 102
    quality of life, 101
    social outcomes, 101
    transitional care program, 102
Chronic medical conditions
  behavioral and lifestyle risk factors, 49
  peer support
    Affordable Care Act, 50
    behavioral health, 62
    chronic care model, 58–61
    in chronic illness, 55–58
    community health workers, 50
    in health care settings, 61
    health information modalities, 62–64
    key functions, 50–52
    role models, 50
    socioecological model, 52, 54, 55
Corporation for National and Community Service (CNSC), 119

F
Festinger's Social Comparison Theory, 134

G
Government Performance and Results Act, 21

H
Health information technologies (HIT), 62

M
Medical community
  Blame vs. Just hospital cultures, 159, 160
  CPPS, 156, 157
  institutional peer support programs, 146
  RISE program, 157–159
  Scott three-tiered integrated model, 167–172
  second victims
    adverse patient events, 146
    definition, 146
    forYOU Rapid Response System, 161, 162, 166
    institutional support, 148, 149
    medical errors, 147
    peer support, 149–155
    SVEST, 172
Mental health
  peer support
    certification and training, 41
    clinician-driven goals, 38
    coping strategies and skills, 38
    funding, 43
    modalities, 32
    mutual peer support, 33, 34, 40
    peer-delivered services, 33, 35–40
    peer-run organizations, 34, 35
    workforce/workplace integration, 42, 43
  prevalence, 31
Mentorship for alcohol problems (MAP), 22
Methadone agonist medication therapy (MAT), 16

N
National Quality Forum, 146
New York State Family Peer Advocate Credential (FPA), 133–134

O

Older adults, peer support
  graphical overview, 116
  patient navigation, 118, 124, 125
  peer companionship programs, 118–120
  peer specialist programs, 116, 121–123
  program types, 117

P

Parent peer models
  Bandura's Social Learning Theory, 135
  barrier-laden service system, 132
  caregiver and familial processes, 138
  child and caregiver symptoms and functioning, 138, 139
  child-onset mental health difficulties, 132
  explicit theory, 134
  feasibility and acceptability, 136, 137
  Festinger's Social Comparison Theory, 134
  key components, 135
  mental health services utilization, 137
  peer-delivered services, 139
  qualifications and roles, 132–134
  Rogers' Diffusion of Innovation theory, 135
  therapeutic outcomes, 132
Patient Safety and Quality Improvement Act, 173
Peers Reach Out Supporting Peers to Embrace Recovery (PROSPER) program, 21
PeerTECH, 123

R

Recovery Oriented Community (RCO), 10
Resilience in Stressful Events (RISE) Program, 157–159
Retired Senior Volunteer Program (RSVP), 119
Rogers' Diffusion of Innovation theory, 135

S

Scott three-tiered interventional model, 167
Second victim experience and support tool (SVEST), 172
Senior companion program (SCP), 119
SMART recovery, 8
Substance Abuse and Mental Health Services Administration (SAMHSA), 6, 10, 17
Substance use disorders (SUD)
  addiction treatment, 5, 6
  community-level support, 19
  criminal justice involvement, 24
  long-term recovery, 5
  mutual aid societies, 7–9
  peer-based recovery services, 3
  peer support, 2
    clinical language, 11
    collegiate recovery programs, 24
    in emergency rooms, 13, 14
    epidemiological research, 10
    high risk communities, 15, 16
    lifelong recovery, 20
    long-term peer interventions, 23
    outpatient treatment programs, 21, 22
    peer based interactions, 11
    peer-based recovery supports, 4, 26
    peer-delivered services, 12
    recovery interventions, 25

Substance use disorders (SUD) (*cont.*)
    in rural area, 14, 15
    social support on recovery, 20
  qualitative approach, 19
  recovery oriented community, 10
  structured treatment, 18
  treatment retention, 16, 18

T
TAPS *Health and Wellness* programs, 79
TAPS *Institute of Hope and Healing*, 80
TAPS *Peer Mentor* program, 78
TAPS *Sports and Entertainment* programs, 80
TAPS Togethers, 79

Telephone Linked Care, 63
Tragedy Assistance Program for Survivors (TAPS), 75, 76

U
University of Alabama Birmingham Health System Cancer Community Network, 125

V
Veterans Health Administration (VHA), 121

W
Wellness Recovery Action Planning (WRAP), 34, 122

GPSR Compliance

The European Union's (EU) General Product Safety Regulation (GPSR) is a set of rules that requires consumer products to be safe and our obligations to ensure this.

If you have any concerns about our products, you can contact us on ProductSafety@springernature.com

In case Publisher is established outside the EU, the EU authorized representative is:

Springer Nature Customer Service Center GmbH
Europaplatz 3
69115 Heidelberg, Germany

Batch number: 08478963

Printed by Printforce, the Netherlands